Atlases of Clinical Nuclear Medicine

Series Editor: Douglas Van Nostrand

Atlases of Clinical Nuclear Medicine

Series Editor: Douglas Van Nostrand

Selected Atlases of Gastrointestinal Scintigraphy
Edited by
Harvey A. Ziessman and Douglas Van Nostrand

Selected Atlases of Bone Scintigraphy
Edited by
Sue H. Abreu, Douglas Van Nostrand, and Harvey A. Ziessman

Selected Atlases of Cardiovascular Nuclear Medicine
Edited by
Douglas Van Nostrand

Selected Atlases of Renal Scintigraphy
George N. Sfakianakis

Sue H. Abreu
Douglas Van Nostrand
Harvey A. Ziessman
Editors

Selected Atlases of Bone Scintigraphy

With 104 Figures in 224 parts

Springer-Verlag
New York Berlin Heidelberg London Paris
Tokyo Hong Kong Barcelona Budapest

Sue H. Abreu, MD
Chief, Department of Radiology
Womack Army Community Hospital, Fort Bragg, NC 28307, USA;
Assistant Professor of Radiology/Nuclear Medicine,
Uniformed Services University of the Health Sciences,
Bethesda, MD 20314, USA

Douglas Van Nostrand, MD, FACP
Director, Nuclear Medicine Department,
Good Samaritan Hospital,
Baltimore, MD 21239, USA;
Clinical Professor of Radiology and Nuclear Medicine,
Uniformed Services University of Health Sciences,
Bethesda, MD 20814, USA

Harvey A. Ziessman, MD
Professor of Radiology, Director, Division of Nuclear Medicine,
Georgetown University Hospital, Washington, D.C. 20007, USA

Library of Congress Cataloging-in-Publication Data
Selected atlases of bone scintigraphy / Sue H. Abreu, Douglas Van Nostrand,
Harvey A. Ziessman, editors.
p. cm.—(Atlases of clinical nuclear medicine)
Includes bibliographical references and index.
ISBN 0-387-97823-2.—ISBN 3-540-97823-2
1. Bones—Radionuclide imaging—Atlases. I. Van Nostrand, Douglas. II. Ziessman, Harvey A. III. Abreu, Sue H. IV. Series.
[DNLM: 1. Bone and Bones—radionuclide imaging—atlases. WE 17 S464]
RC930.5.S45 1992
617.4′7107575—dc20
DNLM/DLC 92-2321
for Library of Congress CIP

Printed on acid-free paper.

Production managed by Karen Phillips; manufacturing supervised by Jacqui Ashri.
Typeset by Bytheway Typesetting Services, Norwich, NY.
Printed and bound by Halliday, West Hanover, MA.
Printed in the United States of America.

9 8 7 6 5 4 3 2 1

ISBN 0-387-97823-2 Springer-Verlag New York Berlin Heidelberg
ISBN 3-540-97823-2 Springer-Verlag Berlin Heidelberg New York

Series Preface

Atlases of Clinical Nuclear Medicine will be a sequence of approximately three to five moderately sized and priced books to be published periodically every one to two years. The series will cover a wide range of subjects, and in each volume typically three to five extensive atlases of different imaging procedures or specific aspects of an imaging procedure will be presented. In some volumes, all chapters will cover a specific organ system, such as gastrointestinal scintigraphy or cardiac nuclear medicine, whereas some volumes will have chapters from several organ systems. The topics of the specific chapters in the atlases will usually include several chapters of current interest and one or two chapters of less frequently performed procedures. However, all of the chapters will be typically directed toward the clinical practice of nuclear medicine.

The purpose of this series is to bring to the reader selected atlases of nuclear medicine, which (1) have never been published before, (2) are more extensive than those previously published, or (3) are more current than those previously published.

The series will be of value to the practicing physician and radiologist as well as the resident learning clinical nuclear medicine. The nuclear medicine physician or radiologist will find these atlases a source of practical information for procedures that he or she already performs as well as for specific aspects of a procedure that he or she is only occasionally called on to perform and interpret. For the physician learning nuclear medicine, these atlases will be an excellent training tool and source of information. Teaching points are emphasized. In addition, other physicians from associated specialties such as gastroenterology, orthopedic surgery, and cardiology will find individual volumes valuable.

The typical atlas will feature an introductory text followed by a gallery of images. In the introductory text, such items as technique (imaging procedure, computer acquisition analysis), physiologic mechanism of the radiopharmaceutical, estimated radiation absorbed dose, visual description/interpretation, discussion, and references will be presented. In the atlas section, each image will have a legend describing the image, which frequently will be followed by a comment section. Although the introduction section may have a significant amount of text and information, the emphasis is on the images, with a significant portion of the chapter's text and information in the legend and comment section of each image. I believe this format will not only help the resident in learning a procedure or a specific aspect of a procedure in nuclear medicine, but the format will also help the experienced physician locate topics that are directly relevant to a particular clinical problem.

Finally, I welcome any comments regarding the series and volumes, and I solicit suggestions for future atlases.

Douglas Van Nostrand
Series Editor

Preface

Bone scintigraphy remains one of the most frequently performed procedures in Nuclear Medicine, and this volume presents atlases of three important areas of bone scintigraphy as well as an atlas of SPECT (Single Photon Emission Computer Tomography) Quality Assurance, which is critical to quality SPECT bone scintigraphy.

Chapter 1. In the past, evaluation of metastatic bone disease has been the most frequent indication for bone scintigraphy, however, the evaluation of skeletal trauma has become a frequent and in some institutions the most frequent indication for bone scintigraphy. In the first chapter, Drs. Siegel, Mandell and Alavi present an atlas of skeletal trauma, which discusses such areas as traumatic fractures, occult stress fractures, shin splints, Toddler's fractures, child abuse injuries, myositis ossificans, non-union, and other traumatic related entities.

Chapter 2. With more and more bone scintigraphy being performed with SPECT, a more indepth understanding of anatomy and a greater ability to identify the anatomy on the images is required. Drs. Gates, Front, Ziessman, and Israel present an extensive atlas of the normal cross-section anatomy on SPECT bone scintigraphy for the most frequently imaged skeletal areas—thoracic spine, lumbar spine, pelvis, hips, and skull.

Chapter 3. SPECT bone scintigraphy also requires more attention to the details of acquisition. The third atlas by Drs. Graham, Lake, and Cohen present a quality control program for SPECT imaging with clinical examples to help illustrate the effects of poor quality control. This chapter includes discussions of x–y axes calibration, center of rotation, parallelism of collimator holes, alignment of conjugate views, field uniformity correction, angular sampling, matric size, and phantoms. This chapter should not only be of value in SPECT bone scintigraphy, but this chapter should also compliment the third volume of this series, which will discuss SPECT cardiac perfusion imaging.

Chapter 4. The book concludes with an atlas that should aid any Nuclear Medicine physician and Nuclear Radiologist who is called upon to interpret bone scans and/or Indium-111 white blood cells scans of patients with porous coated hip prostheses. Although significant data has been published regarding the bone scintigraphic finds in cemented prostheses, these findings do not apply to uncemented prostheses. Drs. Oswald and Van Nostrand present the spectrum of normal findings of porous coated hip prostheses on bone and Indium-111 scintigraphy.

We believe that all or significant portions of these four chapters will be valuable to you in your clinical Nuclear Medicine practice.

Sue H. Abreu
Douglas Van Nostrand
Harvey A. Ziessman

Contents

Contributors

Abass Alavi, M.D., Division of Nuclear Medicine, Department of Radiology, Hospital of the University of Pennsylvania, 3400 Spruce St., Philadelphia, PA 19104 USA

Marvin B. Cohen, M.D., VA Medical Center, Nuclear Medicine Service, 16111 Plummer St., Sepulveda, CA 91343 USA; Department of Medicine, UCLA School of Medicine, 10833 Le Conte Avenue, Los Angeles, CA 90024 USA

Dov Front, M.D., Elizabeth and Sydney Corob Professor of Life Sciences, Department of Nuclear Medicine, Rambam Medical Center and Faculty of Medicine, Technion-Israel Institute of Technology, Haifa 35254, Israel

Gary F. Gates, M.D., Director of Nuclear Medicine Department, St. Vincent Hospital and Medical Center, 9205 S.W. Barnes Rd., Portland, Oregon 97225 USA; Clinical Professor of Diagnostic Radiology, School of Medicine, Oregon Health Sciences University, USA

L. Stephen Graham, M.D., Ph.D., VA Medical Center, Nuclear Medicine Service, 16111 Plummer St., Sepulveda, CA 91343 USA; Department of Radiological Sciences, UCLA School of Medicine, 10833 Le Conte Avenue, Los Angeles, CA 90024 USA

Ora Israel, M.D., Department of Nuclear Medicine, Rambam Medical Center, Technion-Israel Institute of Technology, Haifa 35254, Israel

Ralph R. Lake, M.D., VA Medical Center, Nuclear Medicine Service, 16111 Plummer St., Sepulveda, CA 91343 USA; Department of Medicine, UCLA School of Medicine, 10833 Le Conte Avenue, Los Angeles, CA 90024 USA

Gerald A. Mandell, M.D., Department of Medical Imaging, A.I. DuPont Institute, 1600 Rockland Rd., Wilmington, DE 19803 USA

Stephen G. Oswald, D.O., Chief, Nuclear Medicine Service, Dwight D. Eisenhower Army Medical Center, Fort Gordon, Augusta, GA 30905 USA

Alan Siegel, M.D., Department of Nuclear Medicine, Philadelphia Veterans Administration Medical Center, University and Woodland Avenues, Philadelphia, PA 19104 USA

Douglas Van Nostrand, M.D., FACP, Director, Nuclear Medicine Department, Good Samaritan Hospital, 5601 Loch Raven Blvd., Baltimore, MD 21239 USA; Clinical Professor of Radiology and Nuclear Medicine, Uniformed Services University of Health Sciences, Bethesda, MD 20814 USA

Harvey A. Ziessman, M.D., Professor of Radiology, Director, Division of Nuclear Medicine, Georgetown University Hospital, 3800 Reservoir Road, NW, Washington, D.C., 20007, USA

CHAPTER 1

Atlas of Skeletal Trauma

Alan Siegel, Gerald A. Mandell, and Abass Alavi

Bone scintigraphy for the evaluation of trauma is simple, rapid, and highly sensitive. Although it does not offer the anatomic resolution of plain film radiography, its exquisite sensitivity in the detection of focal functional derangement makes it ideal for the detection of occult fractures, stress fractures, and shin splints. Because it is intimately related to bone turnover and reparation, bone scanning is useful in determining the chronicity and stability of such conditions as compression fractures, spondylolysis, and fracture non-union. Furthermore, its inherent low radiation dose makes this technique a first line imaging study for suspected child abuse. The initial section of this chapter will briefly discuss the technique, physiologic mechanism of the radiopharmaceutcal, estimated radiation absorbed dose, and visual description and intepretation of bone scintigraphy in skeletal trauma. This will be followed by the atlas of skeletal trauma.

Techniques

Bone scans are performed after the intravenous administration of 740 to 925 MBq (20–25 mCi) for adults or 7.4 μCi/kg (with a maximum of 20 mCi) in children of technetium-99m methylene diphosphonate (MDP) or other phosphate bone tracers. Localization into the skeleton will begin within 20 min. About one half of the injected dose will be removed from the background through urinary excretion; the rest will be taken up by bone (in normal individuals). It is preferable to image the patient when the target to background ratio is the highest. This will depend on such parameters as the status of the vascular and renal function in the patient and the half-life of the agent (6 hr) (3 hr after injection is usually satisfactory). After dose administration, the patient is asked to drink plenty of fluids and to return in 3 hr. He may eat in the interim.

The patient is placed under the gamma camera, supine, seated or standing. Using a low energy all purpose collimator, images of the axial skeleton are obtained for 500,000 counts each. The first image of an extremity is taken for 250,000 counts and the contralateral image is then taken for an equal amount of time. Imaging parameters may differ based on the type of camera used. For example, cameras with motor driven heads can image an entire skeleton with automated anterior and posterior passes over the entire body.

If rapid, sequential images are acquired during the initial minute of the study, the perfusion to the area of the body being imaged can be evaluated constituting, in effect, a radionuclide angiogram. This is the first phase of a three-phase bone scan. A static image taken before bone localization occurs will provide a blood pool image: the second phase. The bone scan performed 3 hr later is the third phase.

Three-phase bone scintigraphy is useful for the evaluation of an infectious or inflammatory process, such as osteomyelitis or reflex sympathetic dystrophy. The hyperemia associated with such lesions may aid in their diagnosis.

The radionuclide angiogram is performed by first positioning the area of interest below the camera. A dynamic acquisition of 2- or 3-sec images is performed as the injection is made. The study should be carried out for 30 to 120 sec. Acquisition on a computer will allow the images to be replayed dynamically. The blood pool images should be taken within 20 min; however, it is preferable to begin immediately after phase one. These images should be taken of the area in question in multiple views, at 1 min per image.

Single photon emission computed tomography (SPECT) is a technique wherein tomographic slices of the skeleton can be created following an acquisition made with a camera head rotating around the body. Reconstruction can be performed in the axial, sagittal, and coronal planes. SPECT images improve sensitivity and anatomic resolution. The SPECT images in the Atlas section were taken from a 360° rotation with the camera making 64 stops of 20 sec each. A Ramp-Hanning filter was used.

Physiological Mechanism of the Radiopharmaceutical

The uptake of bone seeking agents, such as MDP, although a reflection of total calcium content in the skeleton, is directly related to the rate of bone turnover or metabolism.[1] These agents are adsorbed onto the inorganic calcium phosphate matrix. The matrix has a greater surface area in bones undergoing a reparative process and in the growth plates of children.[2,3] Additionally, the increased blood flow that occurs in acute fractures also leads to increased delivery of the agent to the fracture site.

Estimated Absorbed Radiation Dose

Assuming an average patient weighing 70 kg, the absorbed radiation dosages from a bone scan performed with 20 mCi of ^{99m}Tc MDP have been calculated using the "S" method.[4] Dosages are shown in Table 1.1

Visual Description and Visual Interpretation

Because image intensity can be manually set, the detection of abnormalities on bone scans is easiest when the lesions are focal. Hot or cold lesions will stand out on the image more readily when the surrounding bone is normal. The lesion should be identified as being one with abnormally increased or decreased activity and then its location described.

Table 1.1. Estimated absorbed radiation dose.

Organ	Rads
Total body	0.13
Skeleton	0.70
Red marrow	0.56
Kidneys	0.80
Liver	0.06
Bladder wall	
2-hr void	2.60
4.8-hr void	6.20
Ovaries	
2-hr void	0.24
4.8-hr void	0.34
Testes	
2-hr void	0.16
4.8-hr void	0.22

Since there are many causes for "hot" areas on bone scintigraphy, its location and relation to the patient's history are essential. Increased activity in joints is frequently due to osteoarthritis, but if the abnormality is in the shaft of a long bone or in the skull, this cannot be the case. A metastatic lesion in a long bone can appear identical to a fracture and the patient's history should help make the differentiation. In some instances, such as separating fractures due to trauma or osteoporosis from pathological fractures due to metastases, or degenerative disease in the spine from metastases, the diagnosis cannot be made by scintigraphy alone. Radiographs of the area of suspicion may give the answer.

Abnormalities causing diffusely abnormal uptake by the skeleton would not be expected as a result of trauma, but may be difficult to detect and care should be taken when reading any bone scan. Since, as previously mentioned, about one half of the administered dose is excreted in the urine, the kidneys and bladder should be visualized on a bone scan obtained at 3 hr. Absence of a kidney must be noted, and absence of both kidneys and the bladder may indicate that diffusely increased skeletal activity has occurred. This is the so-called superscan.

The evaluation of blood flow and blood pool images in a three-phase bone scan is also best when reference can be made to a normal area. Since trauma will frequently cause diffusely increased perfusion to a limb, the contralateral leg or arm should be included in the study for comparison. Be careful that what looks like hyperemia of one extremity is not truly decreased perfusion of the other extremity. The clinical history is essential in these instances. It is also important, when performing three-phase studies of the arms, to know the site of the patient's injection. The placement of the tourniquet may cause hyperemia. It is best to perform the study with an injection in a site other than the arm, or, if necessary, in the patient's asymptomatic arm. Waiting several minutes after placing a butterfly needle and removing the tourniquet before performing the injection may lessen this tourniquet effect. Focal areas of abnormal perfusion will naturally be easier to detect.

Discussion

The Atlas section that follows emphasizes the points that have been made concerning the imaging of patients with skeletal trauma. Cases have been selected to emphasize the remarkable sensitivity of bone scintigraphy such as can be seen with pelvic fractures, stress fractures, and injuries of the wrist as well as the usefulness of these studies in determining the age or active status of a lesion, as in spinal injuries. In addition, the low radiation dose makes these studies ideal in the pediatric age group, such as for child abuse or toddlers' fractures.

Atlas Section

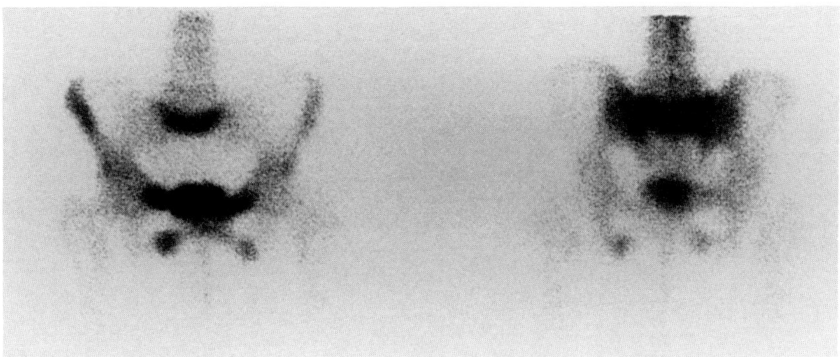

Figure 1.1. Traumatic fractures: pelvis.

A 66-year-old woman complained of right groin pain after a fall. A bone scan was performed and demonstrated foci of increased activity in the superior and inferior pubic rami bilaterally as well as in the S-1 vertebra. Fractures were confirmed radiographically and represented a straddle fracture. In this case, a sacral fracture was also present, but was not noted on the x rays.
Comment: Because of its ease of performance, low associated radiation dose, and excellent sensitivity, bone scintigraphy is frequently the initial imaging study performed in patients with extensive trauma or multiple complaints.

The natural history of fractures on bone scans has been well studied.[5–7] For patients under 65 years of age, 95% of fractures will be positive on bone scan by 24 hr, and almost all fractures will be positive by 3 days after the injury.[5] The acute phase, during which time there is diffusely increased activity about the fracture, lasts up to 4 weeks. Increased activity is well localized to the fracture site during the subacute phase, which lasts for an additional 2 to 3 months. After this, activity in the fracture will gradually decrease. About 90% of bone scans will return to normal in 2 years. Delayed healing has been known to occur in osteoporosis (elderly patients), structural deformity (improper apposition of fracture fragments), and the presence of fixation devices.[5,8] Bone scanning is therefore useful in determining fracture chronicity.

Sacral fractures are often difficult to diagnose by x rays and are frequently associated with other pelvic fractures, such as fractures of the pubic rami.[9] A straddle fracture is due to impact on the anterior arch of the pelvis and can have associated urethral injuries.[10]

Figure 1.2. Traumatic fractures: ribs.

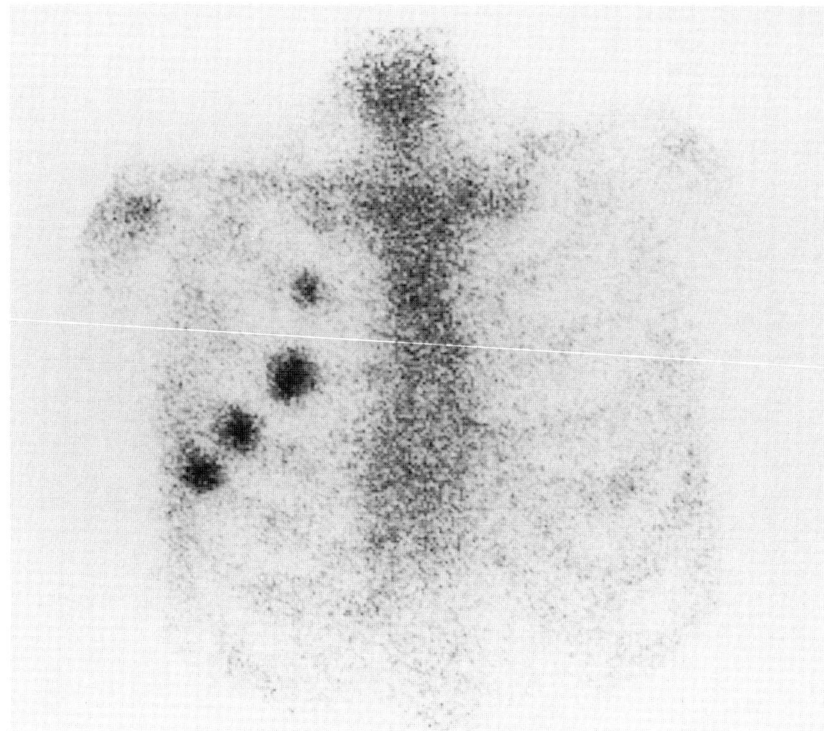

This is a 93-year-old man who complained of pain in his chest wall. To evaluate this pain, a bone scan of the anterior chest was performed and revealed foci of increased uptake in the anterior aspects of the right second through fifth ribs. Note the linear orientation of the four rib abnormalities. A chest x ray confirmed this diagnosis. Only in retrospect did the patient recall falling on his right side.

Comment: The linear contiguous relationship of the four abnormalities is highly suggestive of trauma.

Figure 1.3. Traumatic fractures: thoracolumbar spine.

A 72-year-old woman with a history of osteoporosis underwent a bone scan for the evaluation of back pain. The anterior **(A)** and left lateral **(B)** bone scan images depicted increased activity in the T9, T11, T12, L1, L2, L3, and L5 vertebral bodies consistent with compression fractures. A plain film radiograph **(C)** demonstrated compression fractures throughout the lower thoracic and lumbar spines. The bone scan indicated which compression fractures had an active process: the T11 fracture was the most acute.

Comment: The case demonstrates the typical pattern of acute compression fractures of the spine. Typically, increased activity will be present on the blood pool images when the compression fracture is acute.

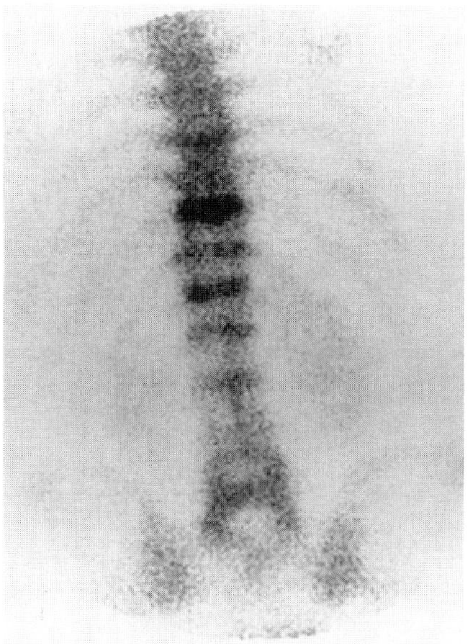

A

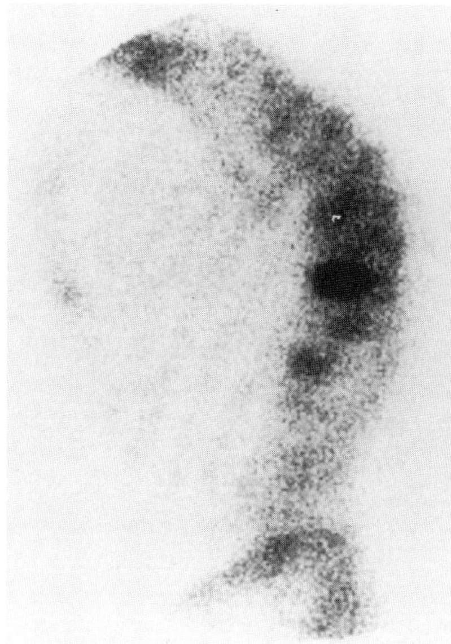

B

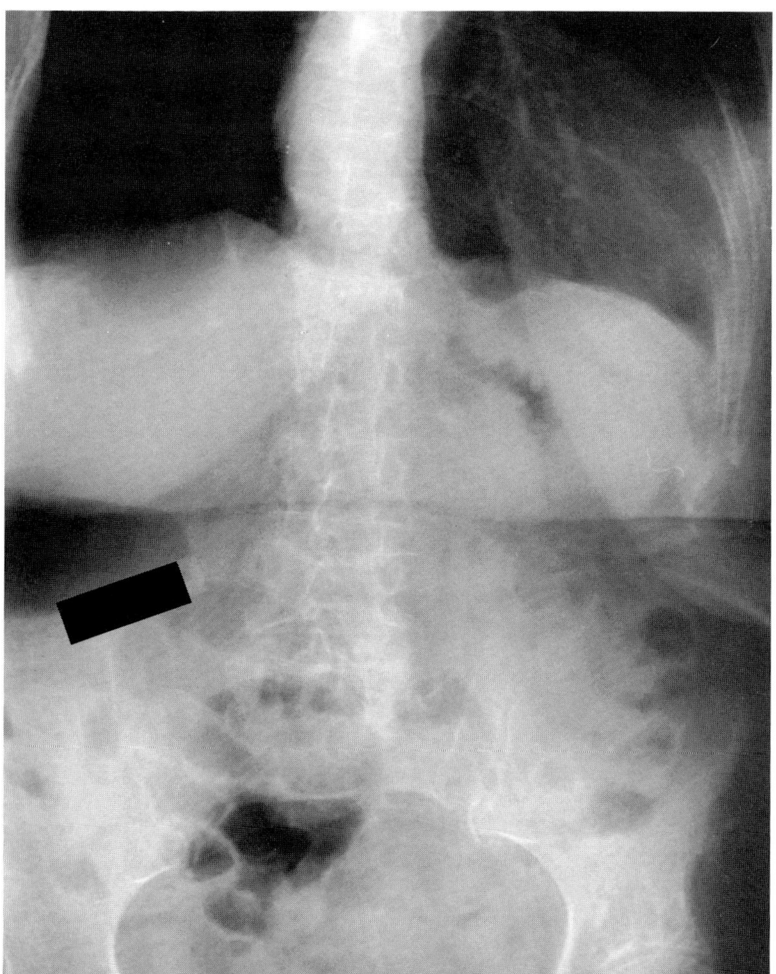

C

Figure 1.4. Occult fracture: wrist.

A 15-year-old boy suffered a hard blow to the right hand. His plamar bone scan image (**A**) demonstrated increased uptake in the distal portion of the right scaphoid (*arrow*) representing a fracture. The normal distal growth plates of the radius and ulna are also seen (*arrowheads*). A radiograph (**B**) demonstrated linear sclerosis (compression fracture) in the distal section of the scaphoid (*arrow*).

Comment: Occult or hidden fractures are usually not apparent on routine radiographs but are readily visualized on bone scintigraphy. These fractures often involve direct blows to the carpus and, in particular, the scaphoid bone in adolescents and adults. The optimum time to initially image is 48 hr after trauma.[11] The failure to show radiotracer concentration at the site of injury 72 hr after the injury would virtually exclude the presence of a fracture in this patient age group. More intense uptake actually is seen in the wrist 10 days after trauma with maximum activity at 3 to 5 weeks.[12] The increased activity at the fracture site in the wrist may last for 6 to 9 months.[13] In several large series of patients with suspected scaphoid fractures, no false negative scintigraphic examinations were reported.[12–14]

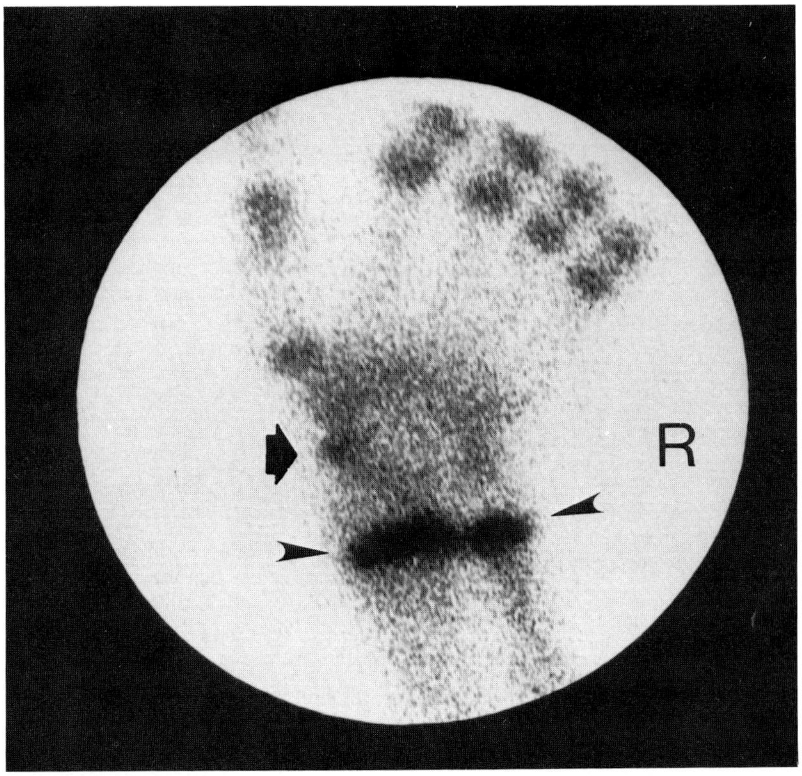

A

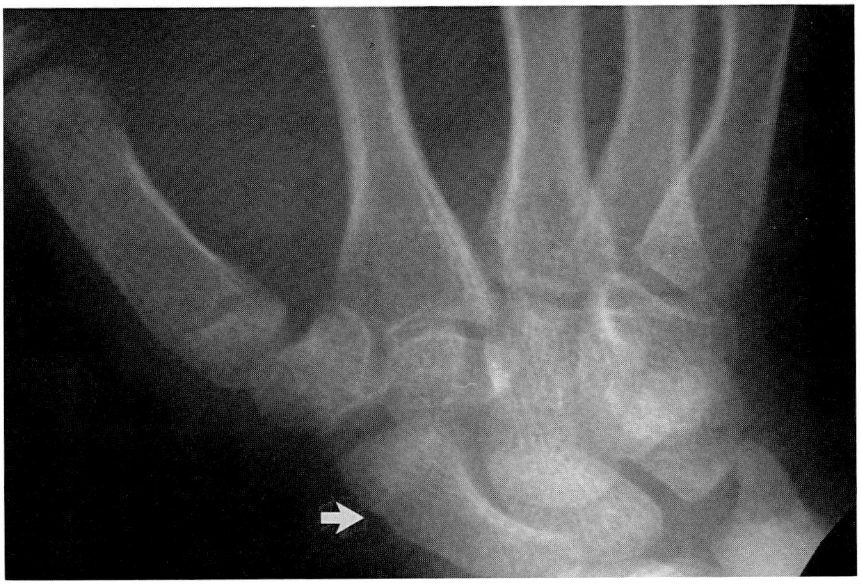

B

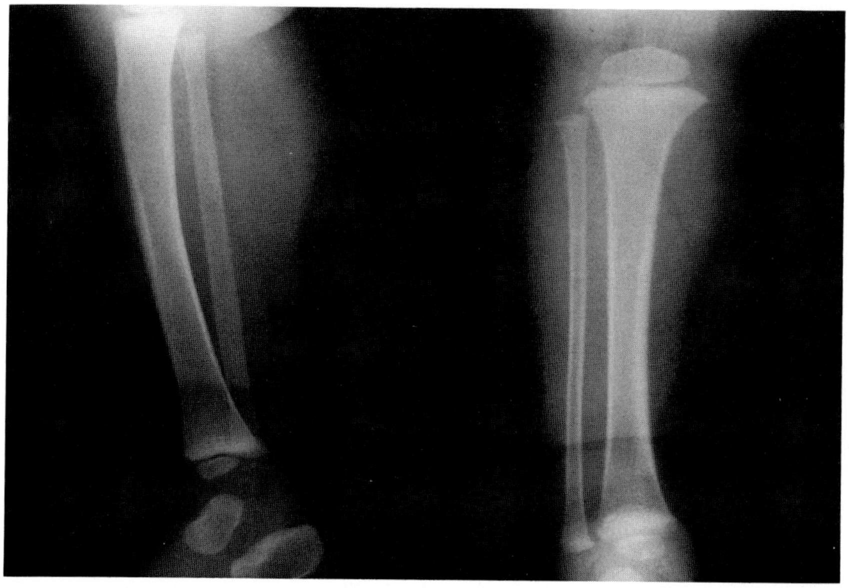

A

Figure 1.5. Toddler's fracture: occult fracture of tibia and fibula.

An 18-month-old male child presented with a limp. Radiographs **(A)** of the distal right lower extremity were negative. The bone scan **(B)** showed increased uptake in the lower two thirds of the right tibia, which is compatible with a spiral tibial fracture.

Comment: A toddler's fracture (spiral nondisplaced fracture of the distal tibia) is the characteristic injury of children 1 to 3 years of age.[11,15,16] Toddlers' fractures of the tibia and calcaneus in young children result from jumping from heights with stressful landings on the distal portion of the lower extremity. The lesion may exhibit focal increased uptake in the distal third of the tibia or diffuse diaphyseal increased uptake on scintigraphy. Sometimes the fracture line extends proximally into the upper tibia. In four children between 11 and 23 months of age, diffuse increased activity occurred in the full length of the tibia even when the radiograph demonstrated only a corner fracture or a spiral fracture in the proximal or distal tibia. In two of these patients the abnormality was focal on the blood pool images and extensive on the delayed images.[17] The activity probably becomes more discrete and focal in patients examined after a week. Diffuse long bone activity, however, is not specific for a toddler's fracture in young children, because diffuse long bone activity can also be seen in osteomyelitis.

Figure 1.5. continued on following page

(Figure 1.5., cont.)

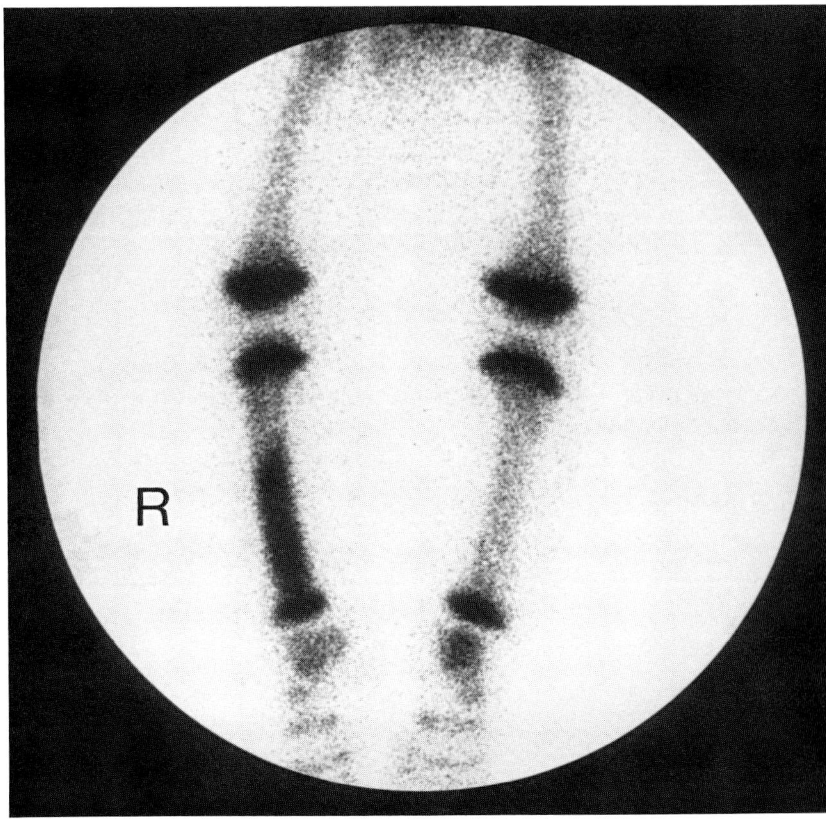

B

Fractures of the long bone such as tibia and radius should be distinguished from "plastic bowing" of the long bone. Plastic bowing or curved deformation of the long bone is most frequently observed in the radius and/or ulna and typically occurs in children after falling on the outstretched hand with the wrist extended. However, plastic bowing has also been reported in the femur, fibula, tibia, clavicle, humerus, mandibular condyle, and ribs in children.[18] In general, applied longitudinal compressive forces of low magnitude cause the long bone to bend. With removal of the transient force, bones can return to normal (elastic deformation).[19] Forces greater than the maximal strength of the bone can cause obvious fractures. Intermediate forces result in plastic deformation or bowing that may persist. Experiments in animals have demonstrated the plastic deformation of bone to be caused by microfractures on the concave side, which disrupt the collagen bundles and canaliculi of the Haversian systems.[20] A force 100% to 150% of body weight is required to produce the deformity. Children's bones are less stiff and absorb more energy before fracture. In plastic bowing, the scintigram shows diffuse activity along the curvature, allowing differentiation of a curved variant from a traumatic bend.[21]

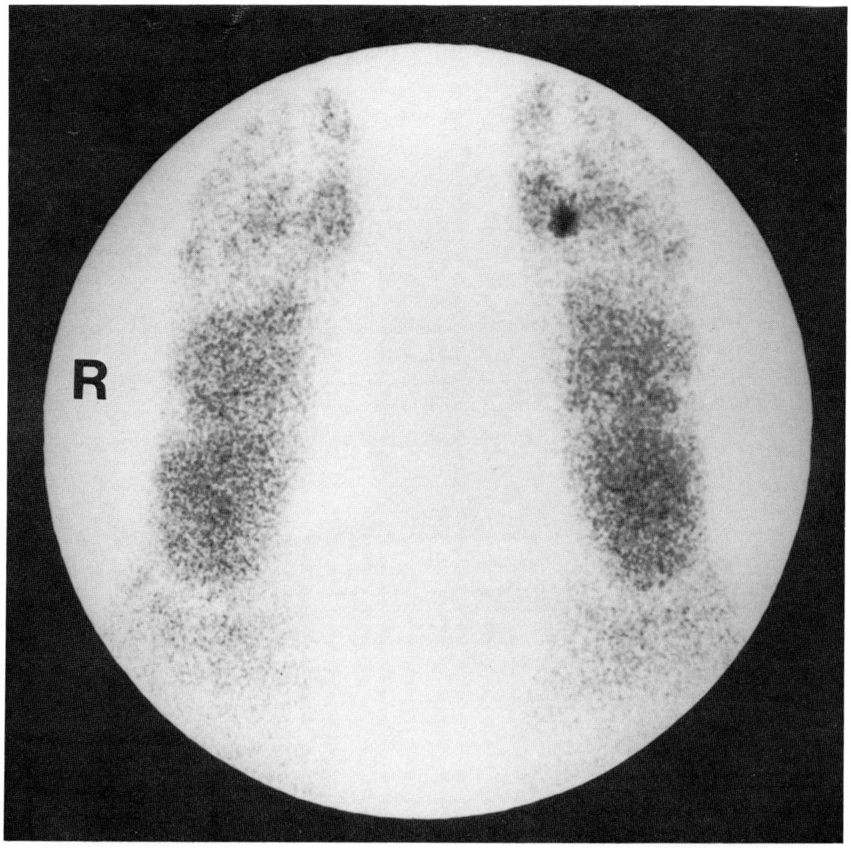

A

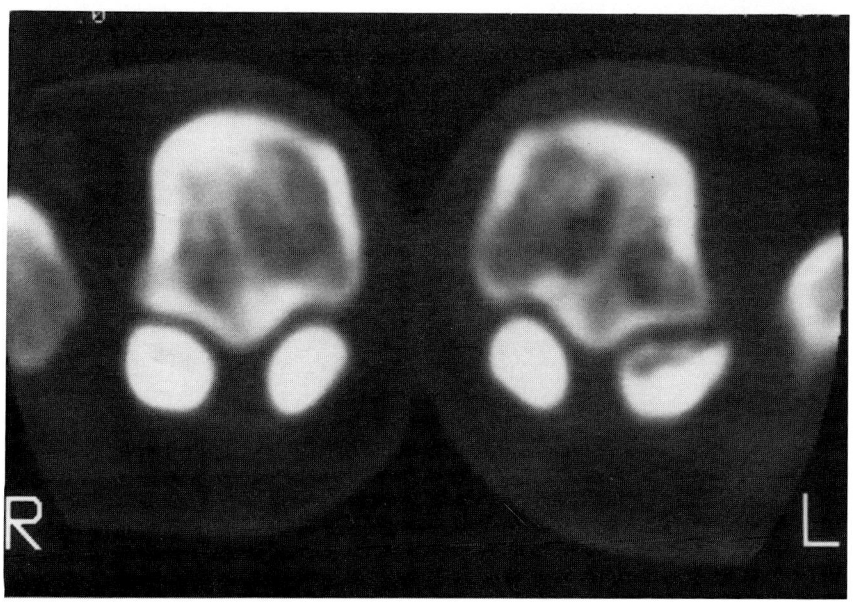

B

Figure 1.6. Occult fracture: sesamoid bone.

This is a 20-year-old woman with two years of pain in the left great toe. The plantar bone scan image **(A)** showed focal increased uptake in the lateral sesamoid of the first left metatarsal. Correlation with computed tomography **(B)** revealed a linear fracture of the lateral sesamoid.

Comment: Due to its excellent sensitivity, bone scanning is well suited to the evaluation of fractures of the sesamoid bones. Radiographic diagnosis of these fractures is often difficult.

Two sesamoid bones are located below the head of the first metatarsal. The medial sesamoid bone tends to bear more weight, and it is this one that will fracture more often.[22] These fractures are frequently the result of falls or leaps wherein the patient lands on his/her feet.[23]

The medial sesamoid bone may also be bipartite, a congenitally occurring variant that may mimic a fracture. Bipartite sesamoid bones will usually be smooth and display an intact cortex whereas a fracture line will often be irregular and interrupt the cortex. Bipartite sesamoid bones often occur bilaterally. When uncertainty exists, a bone scan will usually differentiate an acute fracture from a bipartite sesamoid without difficulty. This diagnosis is important since fractures of these bones will often require casting.

The patella is the largest sesamoid bone. Fractures of the patella may occur after a direct blow or when the forces applied to it by the inserting quadriceps muscle are sufficient to cause structural damage.[24] As occurs with the sesamoid bones of the feet, the patella may be bipartite. This is due to the presence of an accessory ossicle during development that is usually small and occurs in the superolateral portion of the patella. Again, this anomaly is frequently bilateral. At times when the plain film differentiation between bipartite patella and fracture is in question, bone scanning will usually make the diagnosis.

Figure 1.7. Stress fractures: tibia.

An 18-year-old female lacrosse player complained of pain in the left lower extremity. Her bone scan revealed foci of intensely increased activity in the posterior cortex of the midshaft of both tibias (*arrows*), consistent with bilateral stress fractures. **A** is the posterior view; **B** is the left lateral view; **C** is the right lateral view. Incidentally noted is diffusely increased activity along the posterior cortex of the left tibia (**B**, *arrowheads*), indicating shin splints, which is discussed in Fig. 1.10.

Plain films of her lower extremities (**D** and **E**) performed the same week as the bone scan are normal. Radiographs were repeated 1 month later and revealed a healing stress fracture in the posterolateral aspect of the midshaft of the left tibia.

Comment: When force applied to a bone is greater than that bone's ability to withstand it, a stress fracture may result.[1] Stress fractures may be categorized as fatigue or insufficiency fractures.[25,26] Fatigue fractures occur when abnormal stress, such as occurs with athletes or soldiers, is applied to normal bone. When stress is placed on abnormal bone, such as in patients with osteoporosis, an insufficiency fracture ensues.

Stress causes remodeling of bone with stimulation of bone resorption by osteoclasts and bone production by osteoblasts. In the initial stages, bone resorption predominates. A stress fracture is the result of continued stress during this time period leading to microfractures.

Patients with stress fractures may present with pain, redness, or swelling of the involved area. Therapy for stress fractures is to refrain the individual from the offending activity.[27] The length of time needed for healing depends on the severity of the injury. Patients are usually requested to rest for about 3 to 6 weeks. If stress continues, the patient runs the risk of developing a true traumatic fracture.

Plain film radiography is usually negative in the acute phases of a stress fracture.[1,27,28] The films may become positive several weeks into the healing phase of the fracture, but, in some instances, may remain negative.

Figure 1.7. continued on following page

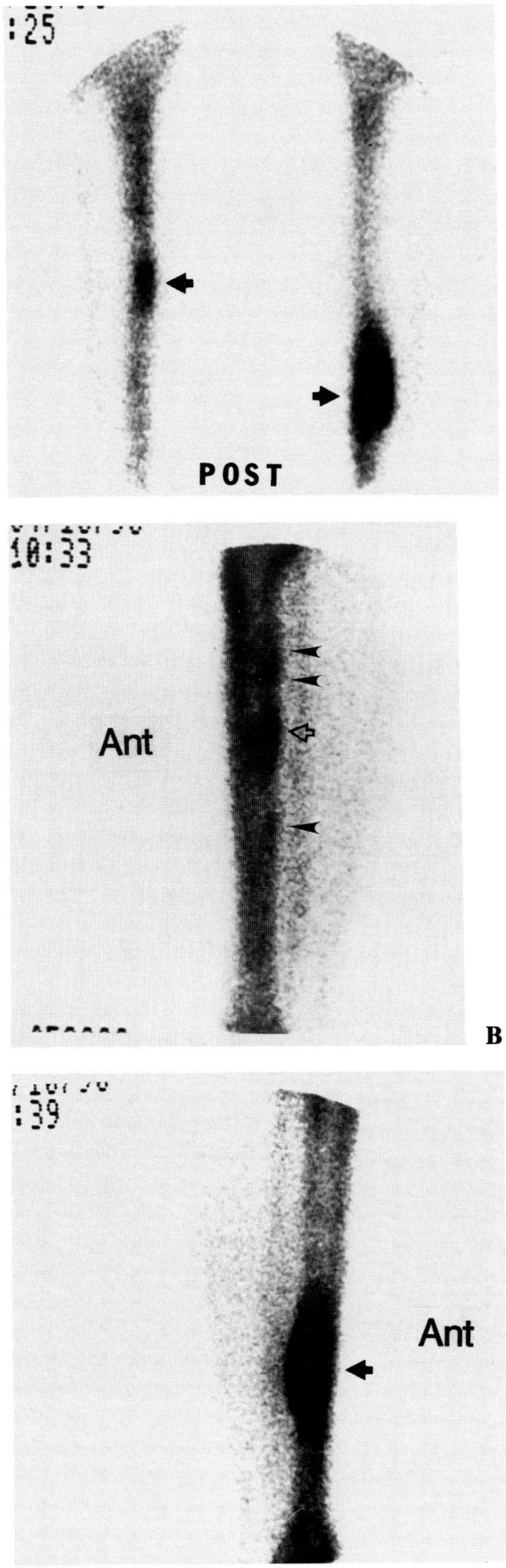

A

B

C

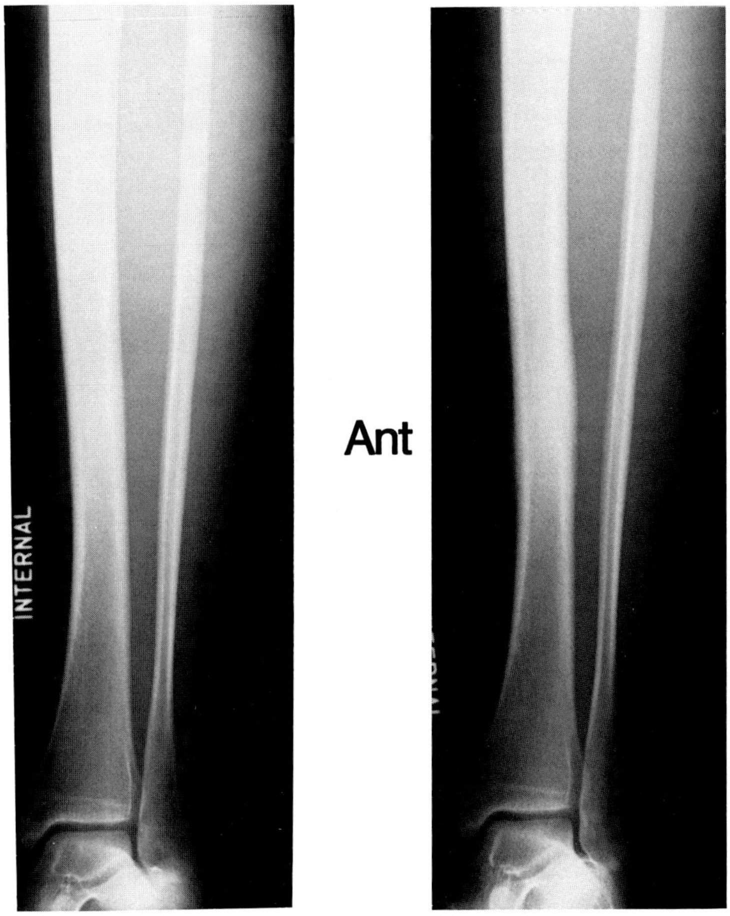

D E

(Figure 1.7., cont.)

Bone scintigraphy is the modality of choice for the detection of stress fractures with a reported sensitivity of close to 100%.[27,29] Bone scans of stress fractures will show a fusiform region of increased radionuclide activity involving the cortex of the involved bone. Several authors have proposed grading systems in which the more severe fracture involves a greater percentage of the cross-sectional width of bone.[1] The acute stress fracture will be positive on all phases of a three-phase study (radionuclide angiogram, blood pool, and delayed bone images).[28]

Bone scanning is ideal for the localization of the injury. Clinically, the patient's symptoms may be misleading. The sites most frequently involved in runners are the tibia (especially the posterior cortex) and fibula (58%), followed by the metatarsals (20%).[27,28] A study of soldiers found the tibia to be involved to an even greater extent (70%). In addition, multiple abnormalities have been found fairly frequently, occurring in 50% of patients.[27]

Not suprisingly, bone scintigraphy reveals that mild stress fractures resolve more quickly than severe ones, with 56% of the mild fractures completely resolved by 3 months and only 12% of the severe fractures completely resolved.[25]

Figure 1.8. Stress fracture: lateral malleolus.

A 62-year-old woman, who frequently walked as a means of exercise, began to complain of pain in her left ankle. Radiographs were performed and no abnormalities were found. The anterior (**A**) and lateral (**B**) bone scans revealed intensely increased activity in the left lateral malleolus (*arrows*), which represented a stress fracture.

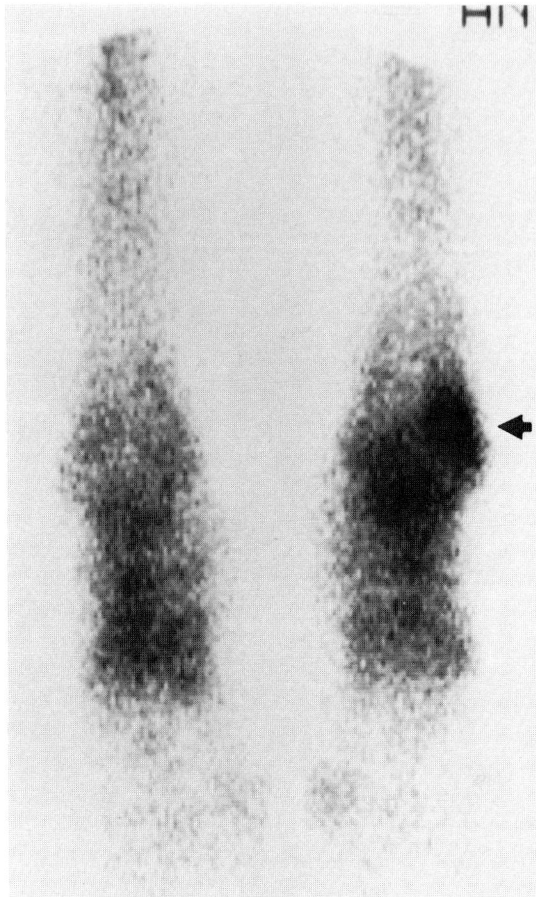

A

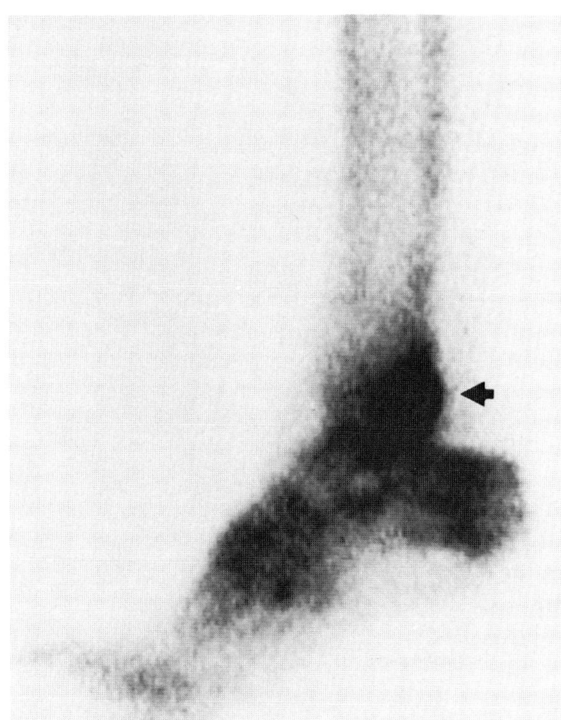

B

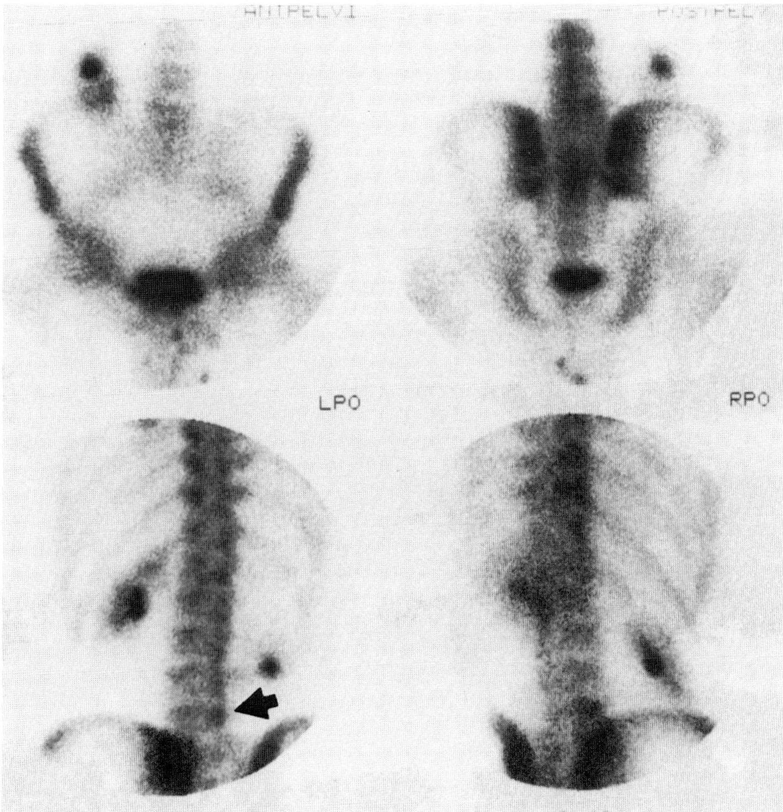

A

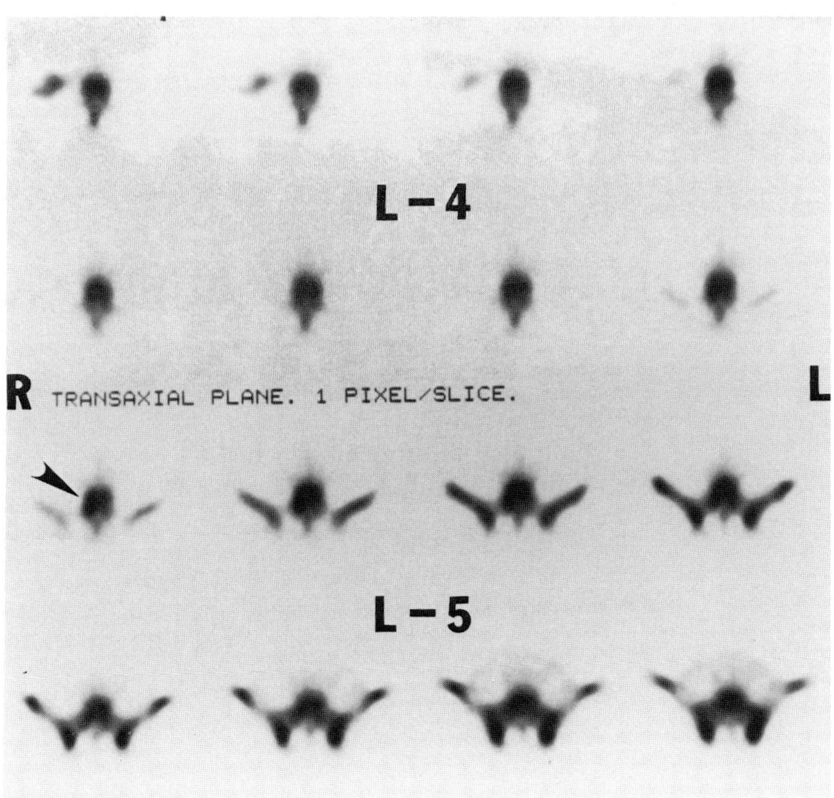

B

Figure 1.9. Stress fracture: pars interarticularis (spondylolysis).

This patient is an 18-year-old man who was active in sports and presented with complaints of persistent lower back pain. Planar images of the lumbar spine and pelvis (**A**, clockwise from upper left: anterior pelvis, posterior pelvis, right posterior oblique, left posterior oblique) revealed a focus of increased activity in the right side of the L5 vertebra (*arrow*). Incidentally noted was a ptotic right kidney. SPECT imaging of the lumbar spine was obtained, and the transaxial view of L-4 (**B**) clearly localized this activity in the right side of the posterior elements (*arrowhead*), a finding consistent with a stress reaction in the pars interarticularis or spondylolysis.

Comment: Trauma to the lumbar spine, especially if hyperextension is involved, can cause a stress reaction in the pars interarticularis.[28] This can result in a stress fracture, a frank fracture, or spondylolysis and, finally, spondylolisthesis.

Bone scans in patients with these injuries will show foci of increased radionuclide activity in the posterior elements of a lumbar vertebra, specifically in the pars interarticularis. SPECT has been shown to be not only more accurate in localizing the site of an abnormality in the vertebra (SPECT is advantageous in separating the posterior elements from the vertebral body) but is also more sensitive in detecting the abnormal uptake associated with spondylolysis.[30,31] The lower lumbar spine is most often involved, specifically L4 and L5.[25]

In patients with spondylolysis evident on plain film radiographs, bone scintigraphy may have additional use. Gelfand et al. examined a series of children with radiographically proven spondylolysis and found about a 50% correlation between sites of abnormality on radiographs and on bone scans.[32] If the bone scan is positive, this indicates that the lesion is acute or still undergoing stress remodeling. When the bone scan is normal, the lesion is most likely old, and the physician should look elsewhere for the cause of the patient's symptoms.[28]

Figure 1.10. Shin splints.

This 21-year-old woman was on the college track and field team and complained of pain in both lower extremities, especially the right. A bone scan (**A** is anterior; **B** is left lateral; **C** is right lateral) demonstrated increased activity diffusely along the posterior cortices (*arrowheads*) of both tibias representing shin splints. Radiographs (**D** and **E**) were normal.

Comment: Shin splints, also known as the tibial stress syndrome, is another form of skeletal injury caused by stress. This entity occurs most commonly in runners when stress is applied to and causes tearing of Sharpey's fibers at the insertion of the posterior tibial muscle, anterior tibial muscle, soleus, or interosseous membrane.[1,25,28] This is not a stress fracture.

Patients with shin splints present with intermittent pain in the legs brought on by physical activity.[1] The treatment of shin splints is reduction of the intensity of the offending activity and administration of antiinflammatory medications.[28]

Plain films are negative in patients with shin splints and, as with stress fractures, bone scintigraphy is the diagnostic test of choice.[28] Delayed bone scan images demonstrate linear areas of increased activity present along the cortex (usually posterior) of the bones of the lower extremities.[1] The first two phases of a three-phase study are usually normal.

Figure 1.10. continued on following page

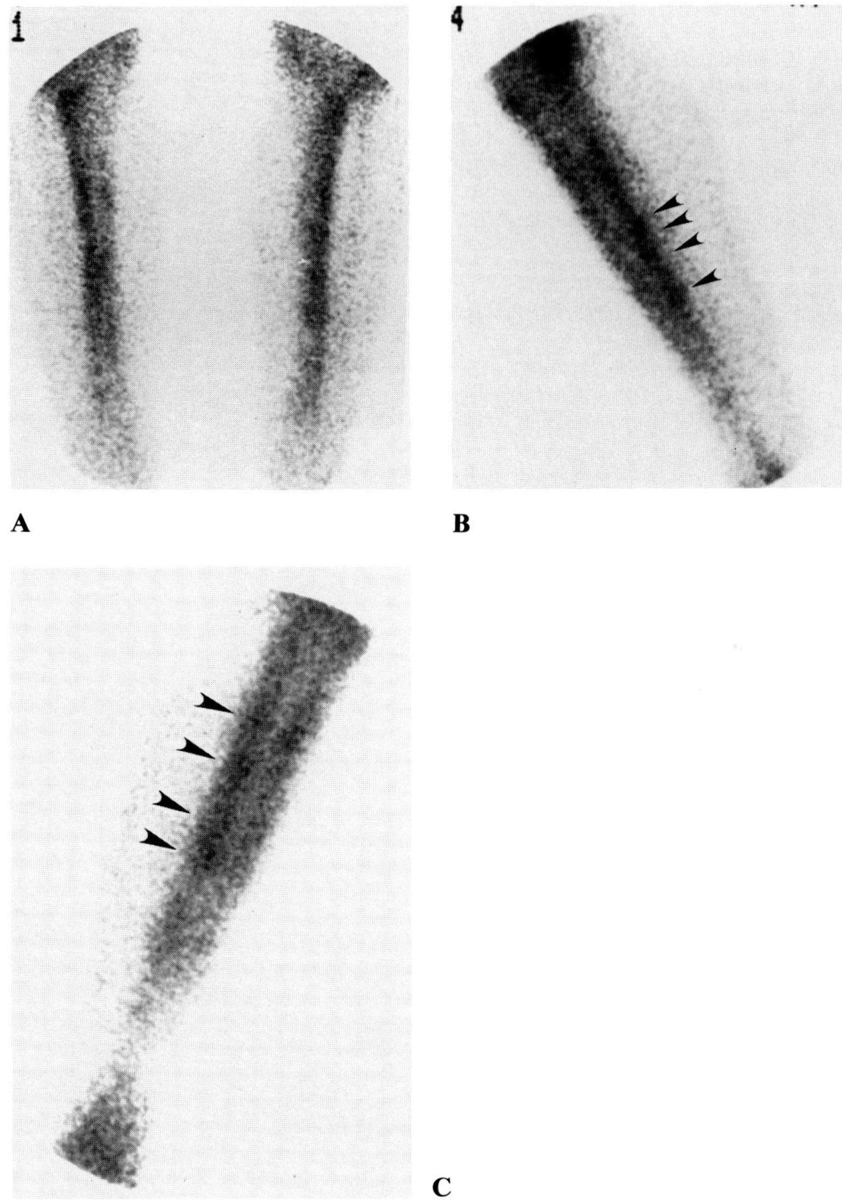

A **B** **C**

(Figure 1.10., cont.)

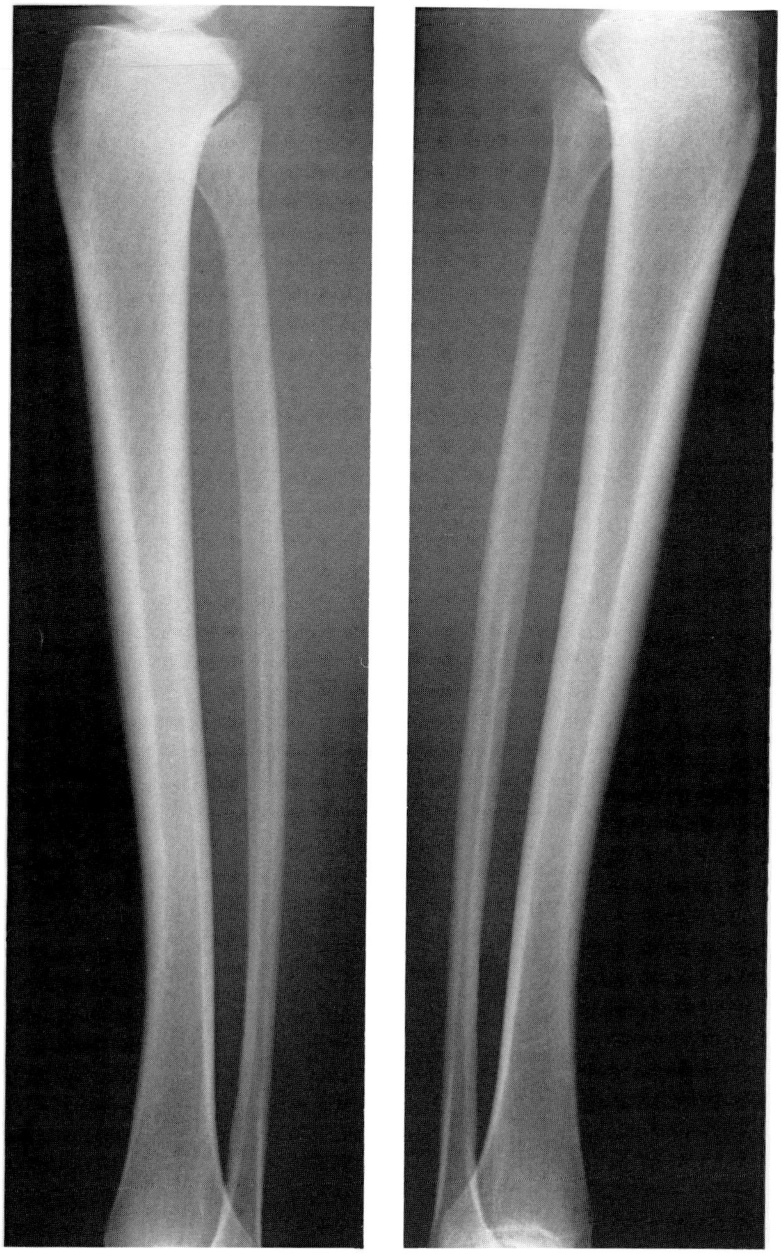

D E

Figure 1.11. Combined stress fracture and shin splints: tibia.

This patient is a 24-year-old female jogger who presented with pain in both lower legs. Her bone scan performed in the posterior view (**A**), right medial lateral view (**B**), and left medial lateral view (**C**) demonstrated increased activity along the posterior cortical aspect of both tibias (*arrowheads*), which represented shin splints. A focus of more intensely increased activity is present in the posterior aspect of the midshaft of the left tibia (*arrows*), which was a stress fracture.

Plain film radiographs (**D** and **E**) of both tibias performed during the same week are normal.

Figure 1.11. continued on following page

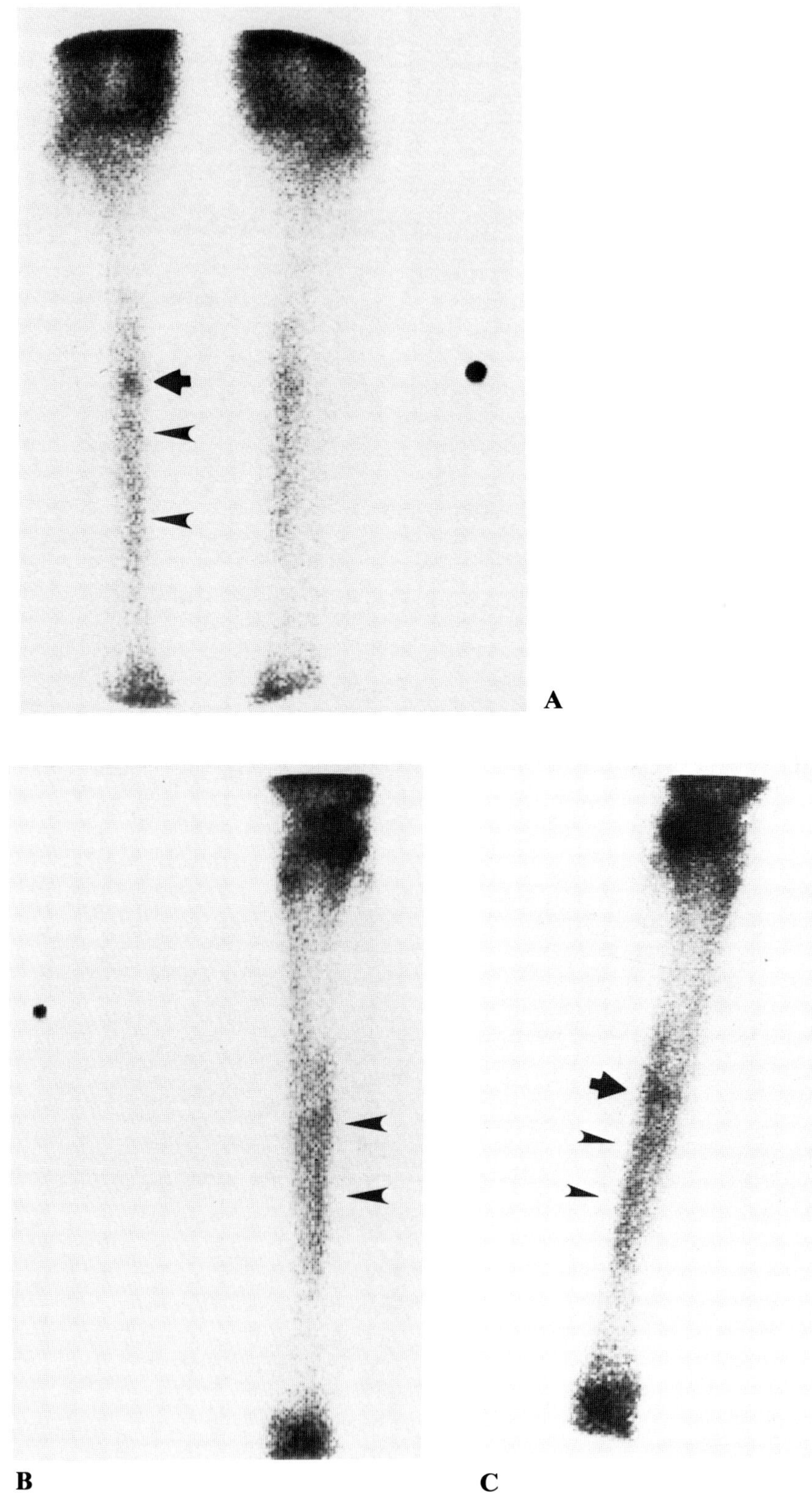

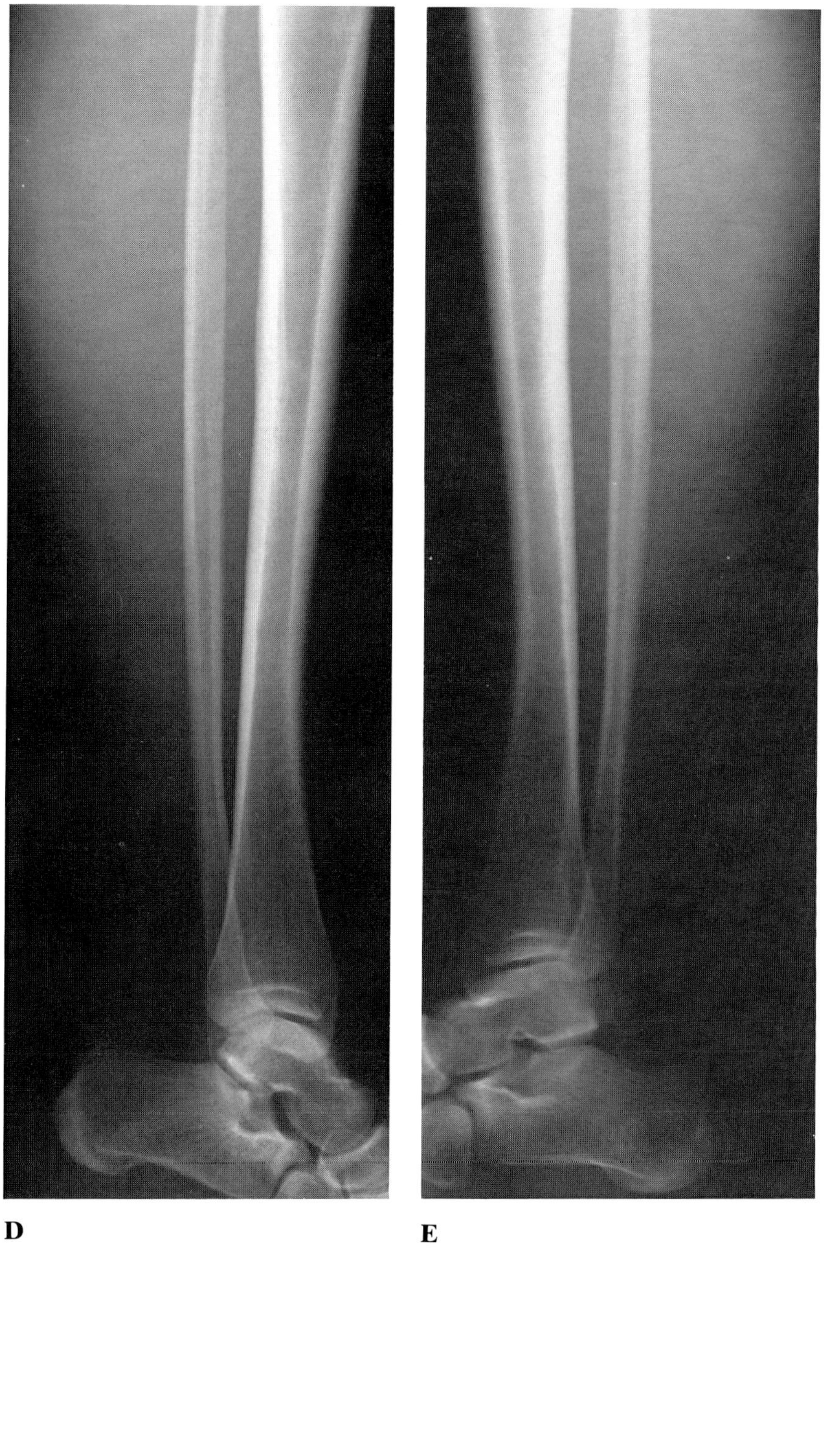

D E

(Figure 1.11., cont.)

Figure 1.12. Combined stress fracture and shin splints: tibia.

This patient, a 21-year-old member of the women's basketball team at her college, presented with complaints of pain in her right leg. Although radiographs of both legs were normal, the anterior (**A**), right medial lateral (**B**), and left medial lateral (**C**) bone scan images revealed increased activity along the posterior cortices of both tibias (*arrowheads*) consistent with shin splints and a more intense focus of activity in the right tibia (*arrows*), at the site of her pain, representing a stress fracture. Increased activity in the medial and patellofemoral joint compartments of the left knee is due to stress-related degenerative changes.

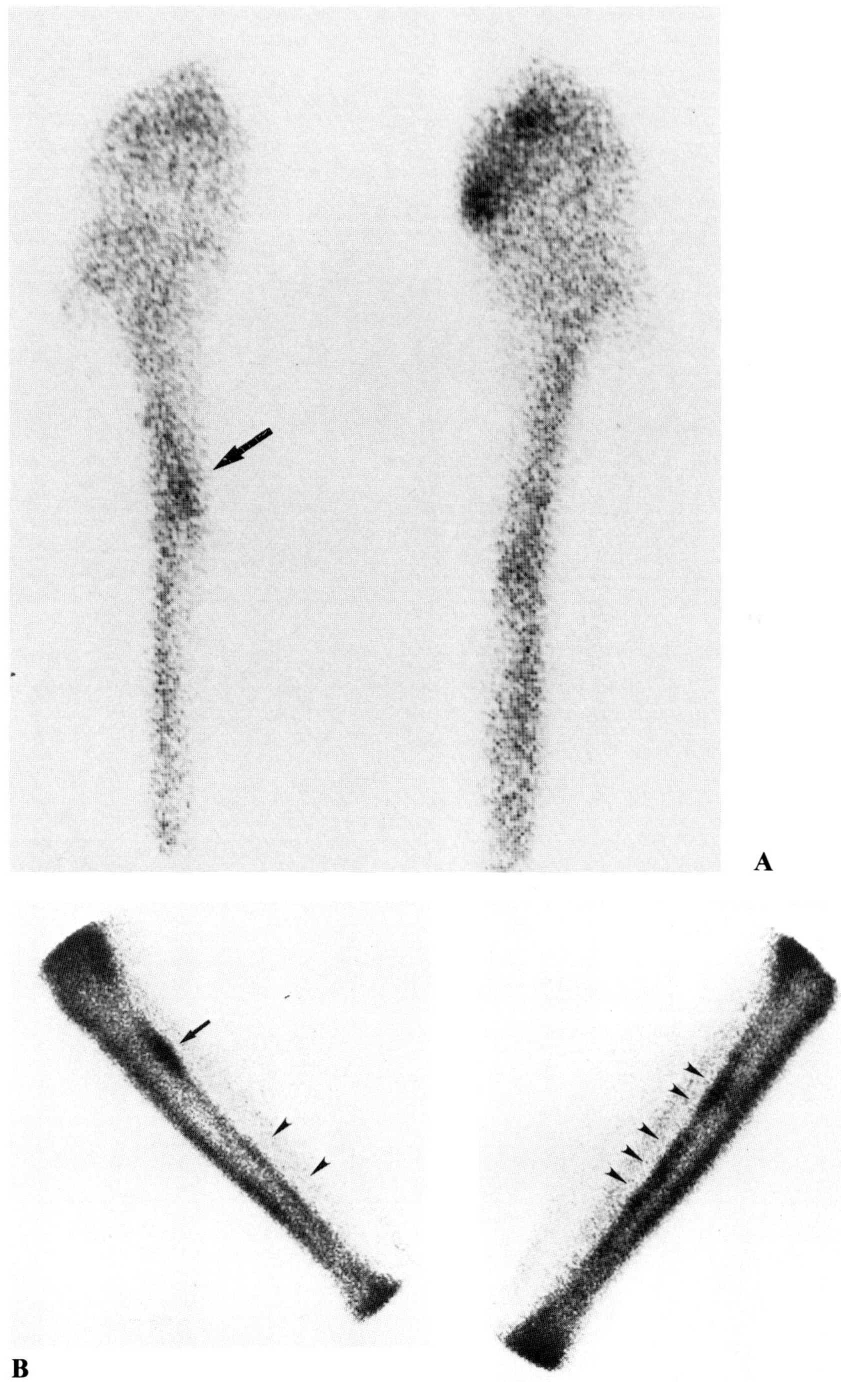

A

B

C

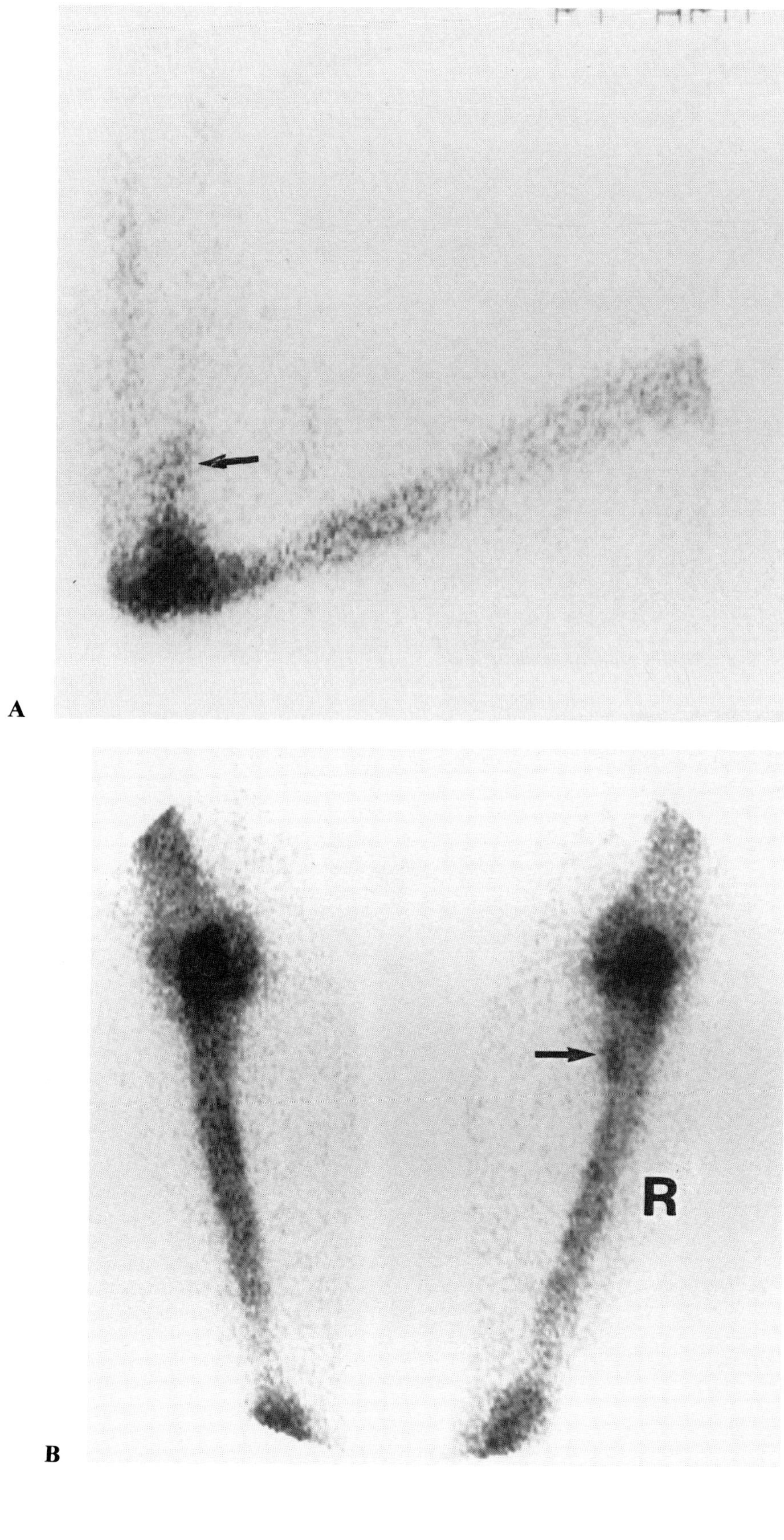

Figure 1.13. Combined stress fracture and shin splints: radius and ulnar.

A 34-year-old weightlifter felt a sharp pain in the right elbow region while bench pressing. Following normal radiographs, lateral bone scan of the right elbow **(A)** and dorsal bone scan of the forearms **(B)** revealed abnormally increased activity in the proximal right radius (*arrows*) consistent with a stress fracture. There is also increased activity in the cortices of the ulnas bilaterally, a finding that parallels that seen in the tibias with shin splints.

Figure 1.14. Child abuse.

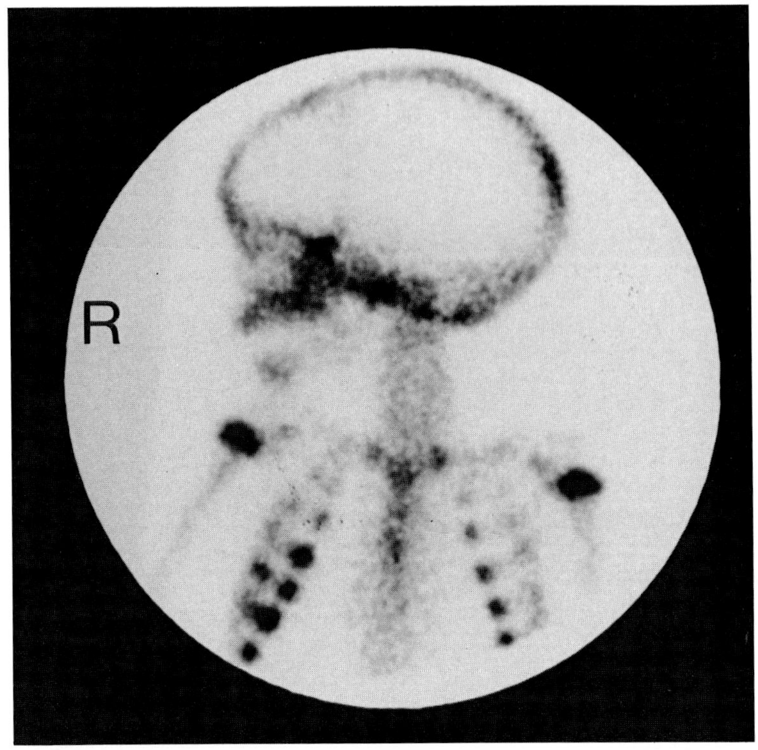

A

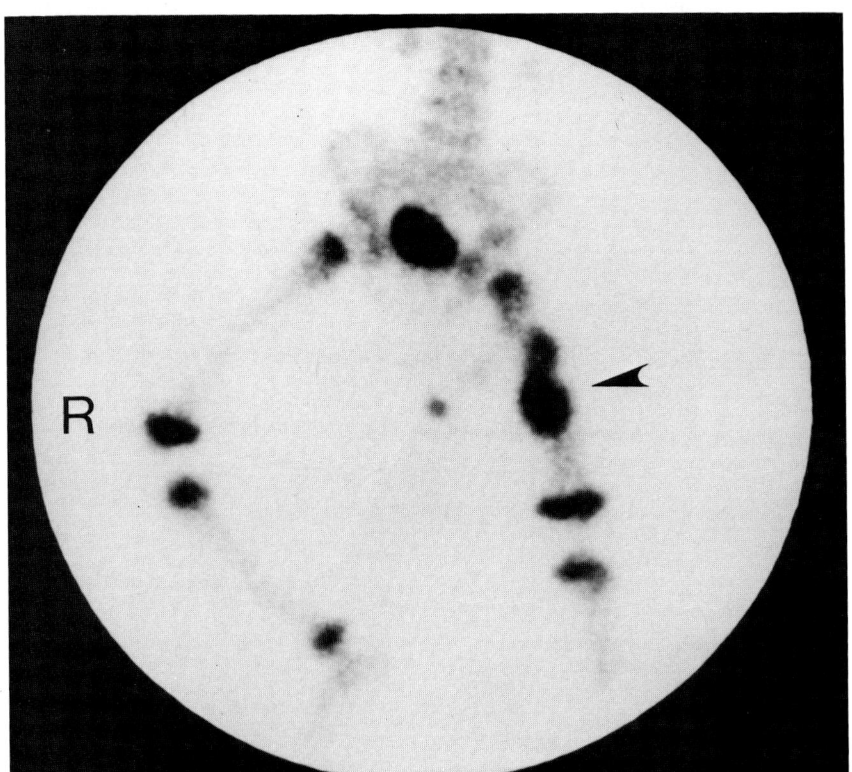

B

This is a 9-month-old child suspected of being the victim of child abuse. The anterior thorax (**A**) and anterior lower extremity (**B**) bone scan images demonstrated multiple foci of increased activity in the right anterior rib cage and mid-shaft of the left femur (*arrowhead*) representing fractures.

Comment: Manifestations of willful assault on children by caretakers can include intentional physical violence, sexual assaults, neglect, and adverse psychological consequences. There is a vast constellation of skeletal abuse requiring radiologic and orthopedic awareness to help prevent the 2000 to 5000 children killed by their parents each year.[33]

Bone scintigraphy is sensitive in detecting early evidence of bone or periosteal injury. Bone scanning can detect the fractures sooner than radiography. Areas of increased uptake can be radiographed selectively. In one series, 50 children had both bone scans and radiographs.[34] Among these children there were 41 fractures. Skeletal survey detected 52% and bone scan detected 88% of these fractures. Both tests have high false negative values. Fractures of the thoracic cage, feet, and hands are easier to detect on the bone scan.[35] Metaphyseal fractures can be difficult to demonstrate on bone scan because of their proximity to the intensely active growth plate.[36] Sometimes pinhole high resolution imaging of the metaphyses will have to be performed. There are reports of the insensitivity of bone scanning in detecting fractures of the skull. Plain radiographs of the skull should be included when the diagnosis of child abuse is considered after a nuclear study.[37,38]

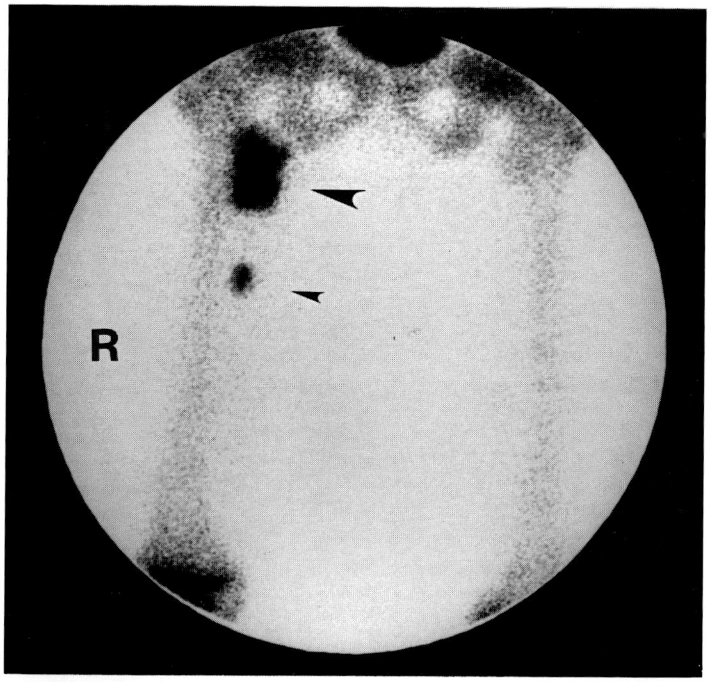

A

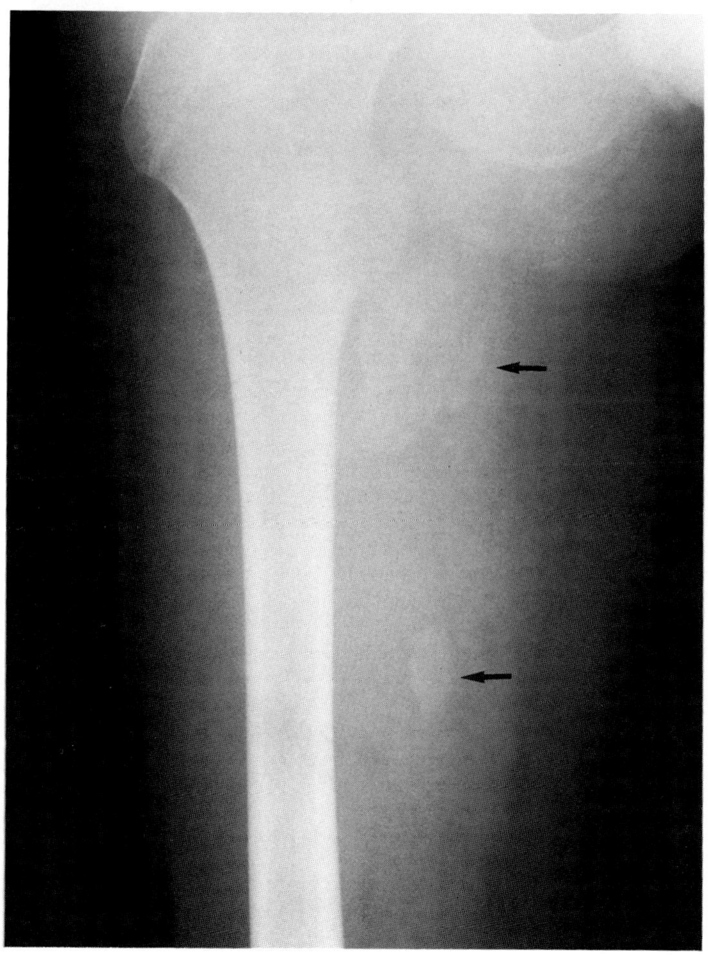

B

Figure 1.15. Myositis ossificans.

This patient is a 15-year-old quadriplegic boy with trauma to his right leg. The bone scan image of the lower extremities **(A)** demonstrated two foci of activity (*arrowheads*) medial to the right femur in the soft tissues representing myositis ossificans. The anteroposterior radiograph **(B)** of the right femur showed two areas of intramuscular calcification (*arrows*).

Comment: Myositis ossificans is the result of muscle contusion wherein calcification, followed by ossification, occurs within the soft tissues. This can lead to pain secondary to increased compartment pressures or direct irritation of adjacent tissues.[28]

The treatment of myositis ossificans is frequently surgical excision. There is, however, a significant incidence of recurrence if this area of ectopic ossification is removed before it is fully mature. Bone scanning is a sensitive way to detect maturation: areas of ossification undergoing growth are metabolically active and will be visualized during scanning with ^{99m}Tc MDP. When fully mature, the radionuclide will no longer be picked up, but the area of ossification may develop bone marrow, which may be detected by bone marrow imaging with ^{99m}Tc sulfur colloid.

Figure 1.16. Reflex sympathetic dystrophy.

This patient is a 47-year-old man who suffered an automobile accident several months before this study was performed. He had persistent complaints of pain in his right arm, especially in his hand.

A three-phase bone scan was performed. **A** and **B** are the flow and blood pool studies of both hands in the palmar view, respectively. **C** is the delayed bone phase images of both hands in the palmar and dorsal views. The marker represents the right side. Increased perfusion and blood pool activity is present in the distal right extremity. In the delayed bone phase images, diffusely increased activity is seen throughout the right hand, especially in the periarticular regions. These findings represent reflex sympathetic dystrophy.

Comment: Reflex sympathetic dystrophy is a syndrome that includes pain, swelling, vasomotor instability, and dystrophic skin changes of the involved extremity.[39] Although trauma is frequently cited as the etiology of reflex sympathetic dystrophy, as many as 35% of patients will present with no specific causative event.[40] Other potential causes of reflex sympathetic dystrophy are infection, peripheral neuropathy, central nervous system diseases, cervical osteoarthritis, and myocardial infarction.[41] The exact cause is not understood.

Plain film radiographs may reveal patchy osteoporosis, especially in a periarticular distribution.[39] This, however, is not a specific or sensitive finding. Studies have shown osteoporosis to be present in only 30% to 70% of cases of reflex sympathetic dystrophy and similar patterns to be present in disuse.[39,42,43]

Kozin et al. indicate that bone scintigraphy, which has about an equal sensitivity to plain film radiography in the detection of reflex sympathetic dystrophy, will add to the specificity.[39] Patients with acute reflex sympathetic dystrophy will frequently have increased blood flow and blood pool activity in the first two phases of a three-phase bone scan. There is increased activity throughout the involved extremity, especially in the periarticular regions, on the delayed image (third phase).

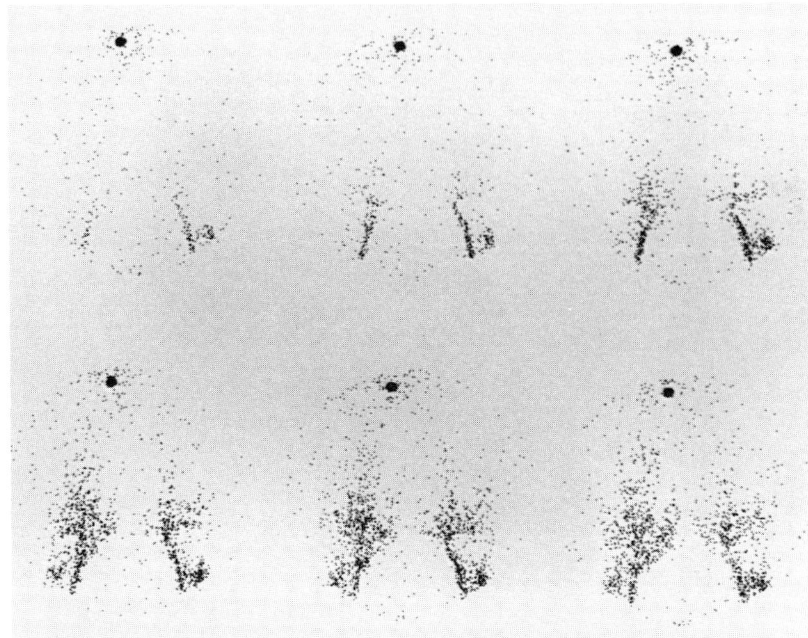

A

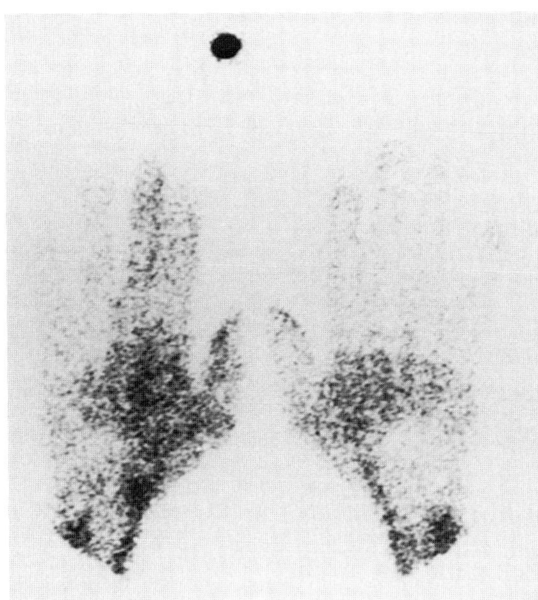

B

Figure 1.16. continued on following page

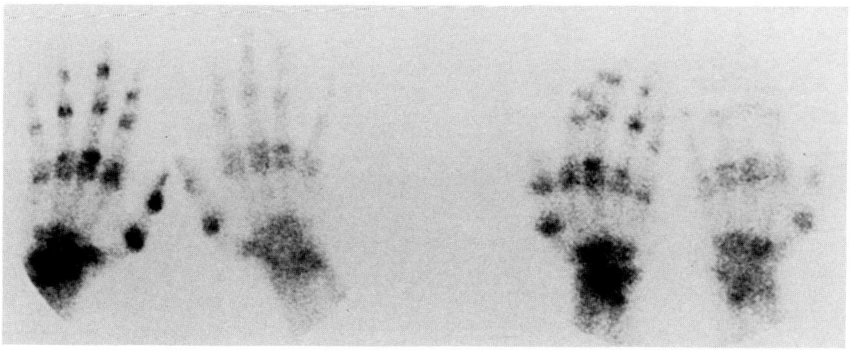

C

(Figure 1.16., cont.)

Demangeat et al., studying reflex sympathetic dystrophy of the hand, have identified different stages of reflex sympathetic dystrophy.[44] Patients with the first stage, which occurs for about the first 20 weeks, have increased activity on all three phases of the bone scan. In stage II, which lasts from about 20 to 60 weeks, the first two phases become normal but the delayed images continue to depict increased activity. Finally, in stage III, the third phase becomes normal but the blood flow and blood pool activity is decreased. This stage occurs from about 60 to 100 weeks.

Furthermore, it should be recognized that reflex sympathetic dystrophy may appear quite different in the pediatric population.[45] These patients may present with decreased activity on the blood flow, blood pool, and delayed bone scan images.

Figure 1.17. Reflex sympathetic dystrophy.

A 62-year-old woman complained of pain and mild swelling of her right ankle. She related no definite history of trauma and radiographs were normal.

The three-phase bone scan is positive on all three phases, with increased flow, blood pool, and bone scan activity in the right distal extremity, especially in the right ankle, all consistent with reflex sympathetic dystrophy. **A** is the flow to the feet in the anterior view, **B** is the blood pool in the feet and knees in the anterior view, and **C** is the bone scan (clockwise from upper left: anterior knees, posterior knees, lateral right foot, and anterior feet). There are also degenerative changes in the right knee. The marker represents the right side.

Figure 1.17. continued on following page

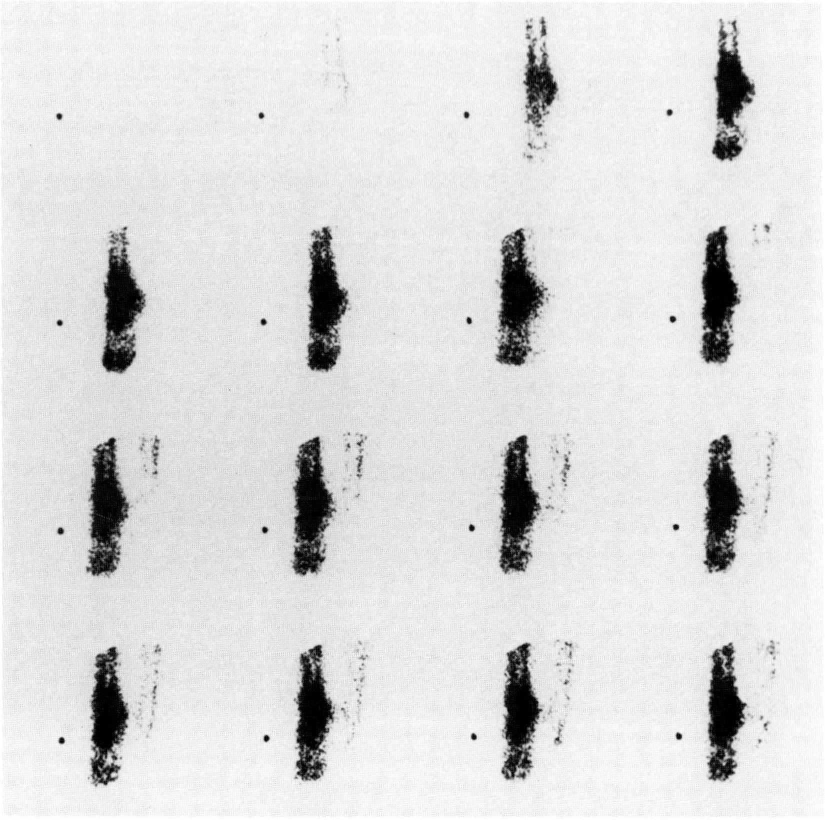

A

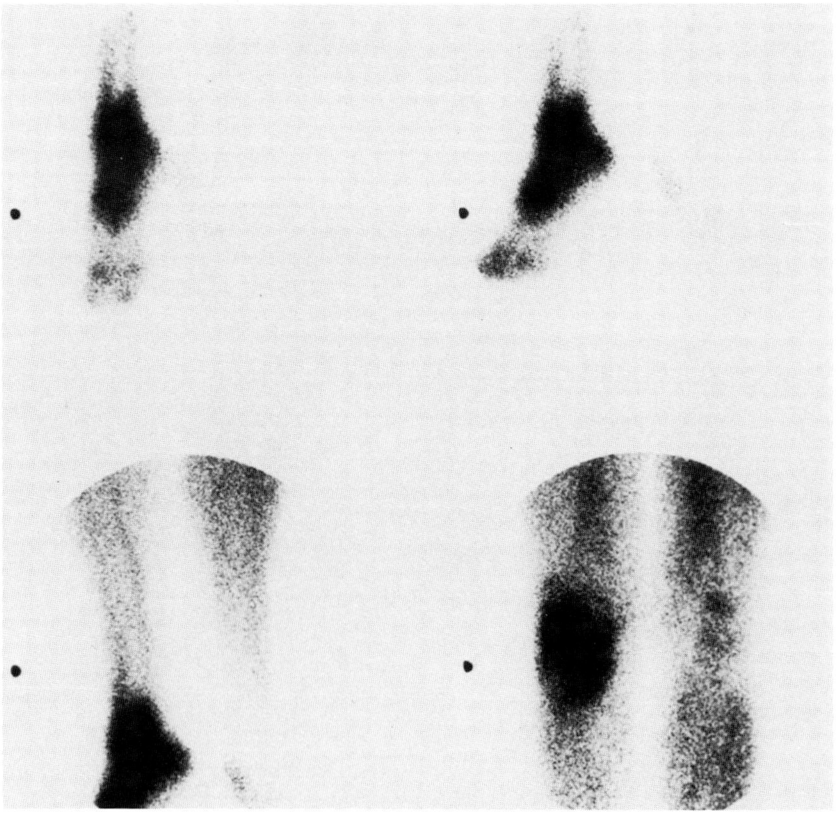

B

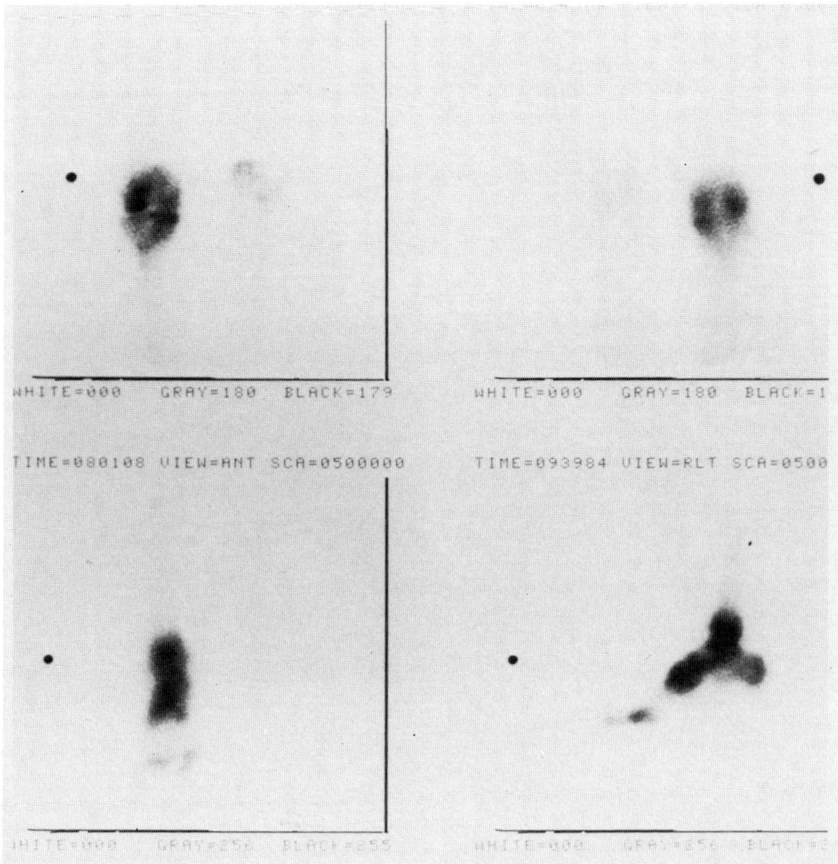

C

(Figure 1.17., cont.)

Figure 1.18. Non-union and pseudarthroses.

This patient sustained a fracture of the shaft of the right humerus and underwent internal fixation of the fracture fragments. After poor healing of the fracture, bone scintigraphy (**A**) was performed and revealed an oblique photopenic cleft (*open arrow*) identifying this as a pseudarthrosis. **B** is the anteroposterior radiograph of the right humerus.

Comment: Fracture fragments may fail to repair within a normal time course (6–8 months) or may never heal completely without surgical intervention.[46] They may reach fibrous but not skeletal union or may develop a synovial lined cavity (pseudarthrosis). There are numerous causes of non-union and pseudarthroses, including infection, ischemia, osteoporosis, hyperparathyroidism, malnutrition, and poor alignment of the fracture fragments.[47] Approximately 5% of fractures will result in non-union.[48]

The scintigraphic appearance of non-union has been divided into three categories, each with a significantly different prognosis for patients undergoing electrical stimulation therapy.[49–51] Patients who have intensely increased activity in the fracture site have reactive non-union fall into Group I and have a good prognosis. If a photon-deficient gap, which would be characteristic of a pseudarthrosis, can be visualized, the healing rate is poor. These patients are classified as Group II. Finally, fractures with poor uptake of activity or uncertainty about the presence of a photopenic gap are called indeterminate or Group III.

(Reprinted with permission from Mandell GA, Alavi A: Scintigraphic evaluation of bone trauma. In Bone Scintigraphy, Silberstein T (ed), Futura Publishing Co. 1984.)

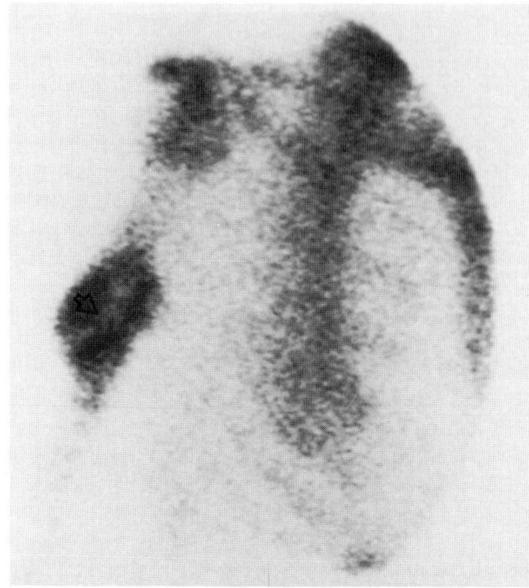

A

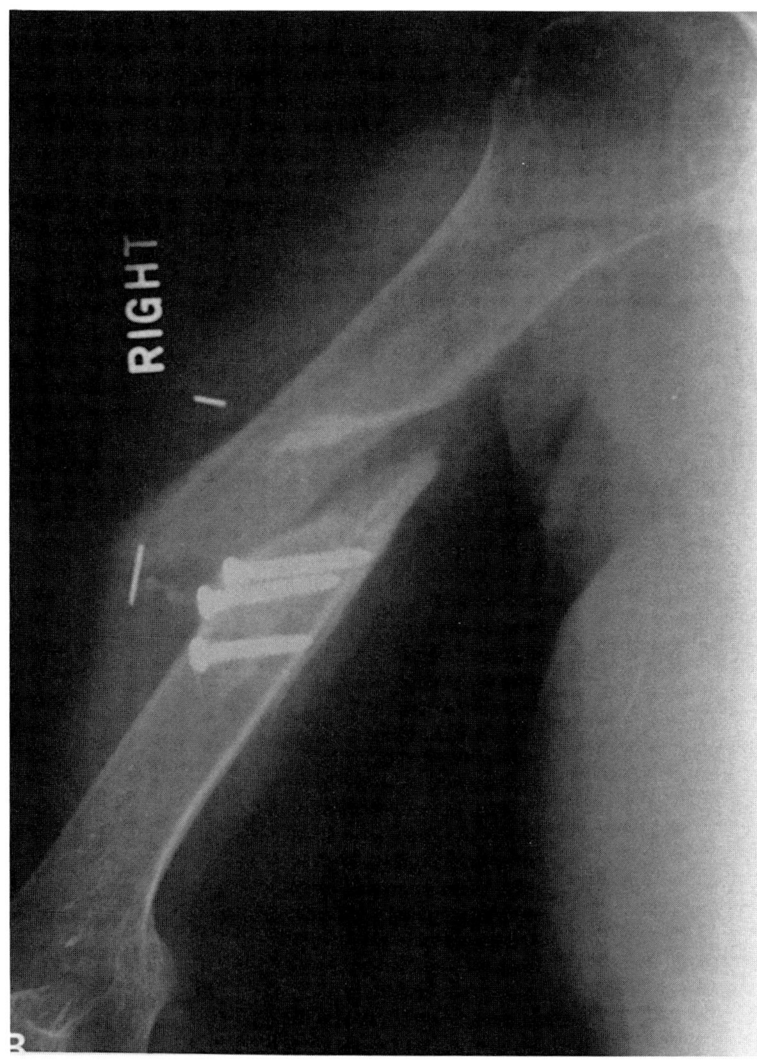

B

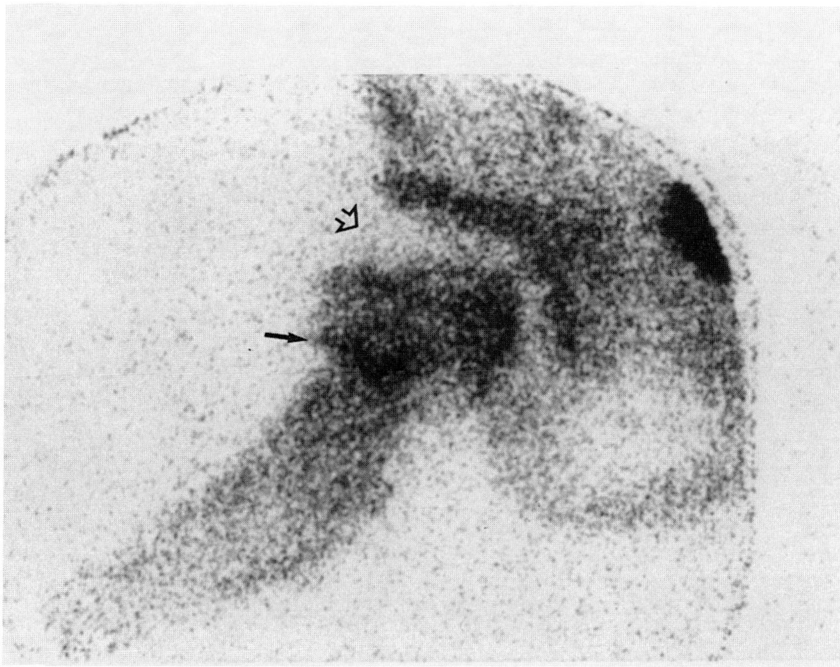

A

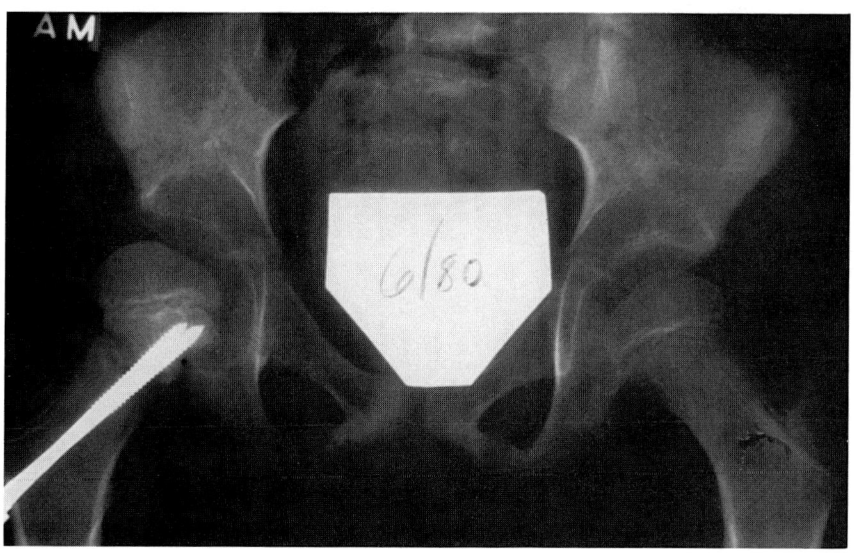

B

Figure 1.19. Avascular necrosis.

A 4-year-old child suffered a forceful blow to the right hip. The anterolateral pinhole magnification bone scan image of the right proximal femur (**A**) showed a photopenic defect in the lateral, superior aspect of the right proximal femoral epiphysis (*open arrow*), indicative of avascular necrosis. There was also medial displacement of the femoral head in its relationship to the femoral neck. A linear area of activity in the right femoral neck (*arrow*) represented the fracture. The radiograph (**B**) showed postoperative pinning and reposition of the formerly displaced fracture of the right femoral neck. The femoral head appeared normal.

Comment: Avascular necrosis (AVN), due to interruption of the blood supply, is a potential complication of trauma. This is especially common in the scaphoid bone and femoral head.

In the initial phase of AVN, the involved site will be photon deficient. Due to proximity of the acute fracture, visualization of this defect can be difficult, and pinhole views may be beneficial.[52,53] Shortly thereafter, the reparative process will begin and the involved site will revert to increased activity before returning to normal.

Figure 1.20. Osgood-Schlatter disease.

A 13-year-old boy underwent a bone scan to determine the cause of his left knee pain. In this three-phase bone scan, hyperemia in the region of the tibial tubercle in the proximal left tibia was demonstrated on both the anterior vascular images of the knees (**A**) and the lateral blood pool images of the left knee (**B**; *arrows*). The lateral delayed image of the left knee (**C**; *arrow*) and the lateral delayed image of the right knee (**D**) demonstrated activity in the infrapatellar tendon and tibial tubercle of the left leg, probably related to calcification in these regions.

Comment: In Osgood-Schlatter disease, the infrapatellar insertion into the tibial tuberosity becomes painful and swollen secondary to repeated trauma in the pubertal or adolescent child. The characteristic lesion results from tearing of the fibers of the patellar tendon. The abnormality is reported to be more common in boys than girls (7 : 1), but with the evolution of more girls participating in similar sports, the male predominance is changing.

The developing ossification center of the tibial tubercle appears unable to withstand the shearing forces and abnormal stresses applied to the patellar tendon resulting in avulsion of portions of the center.[54] The process can be unilateral or bilateral.

Imaging of the knee in Osgood-Schlatter disease should be obtained only when symptoms or signs are atypical. Soft tissue swelling of the patellar tendon is the most frequent radiographic finding of acute disease. Irregular ossification can occasionally be visualized at the attachment of the tendon at the tibial tubercle. When the symptoms are not compatible with Osgood-Schlatter disease and plain radiography does not disclose any other etiology, a bone scan may be necessary. The mechanism of deposition of the radiopharmaceutical in the infrapatellar tendon is not known but probably depends on hyperemia and microscopic calcification of the tendon.

Figure 1.20. continued on following page

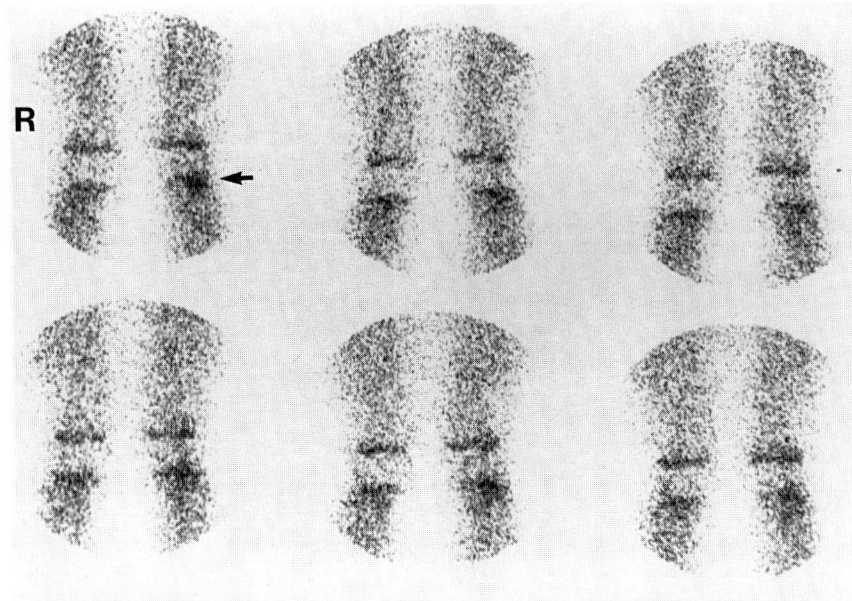

A

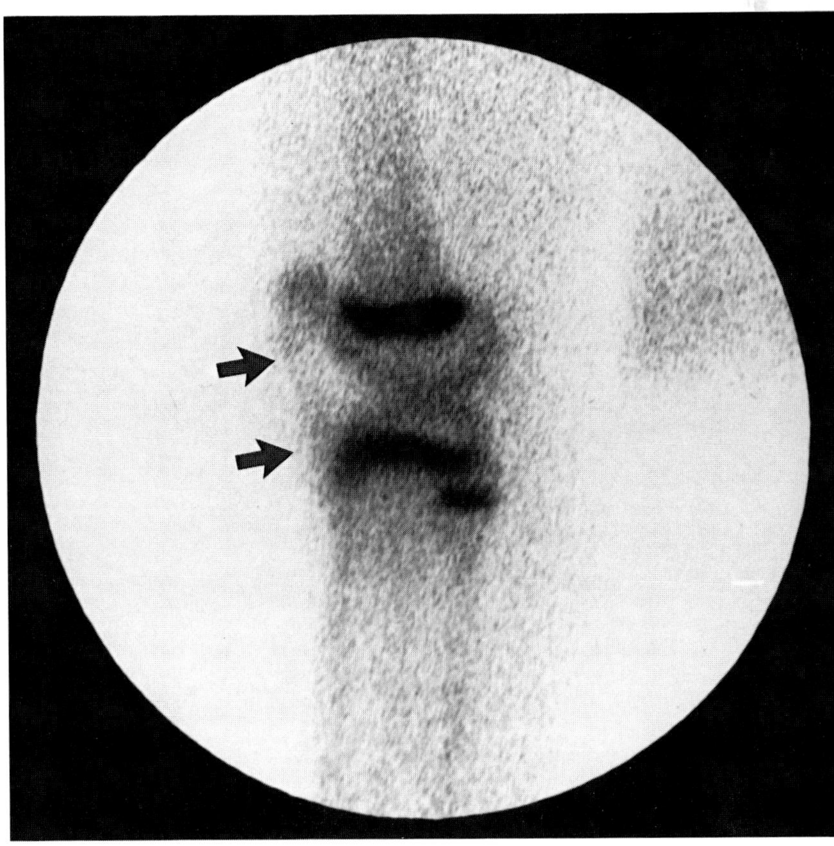

B

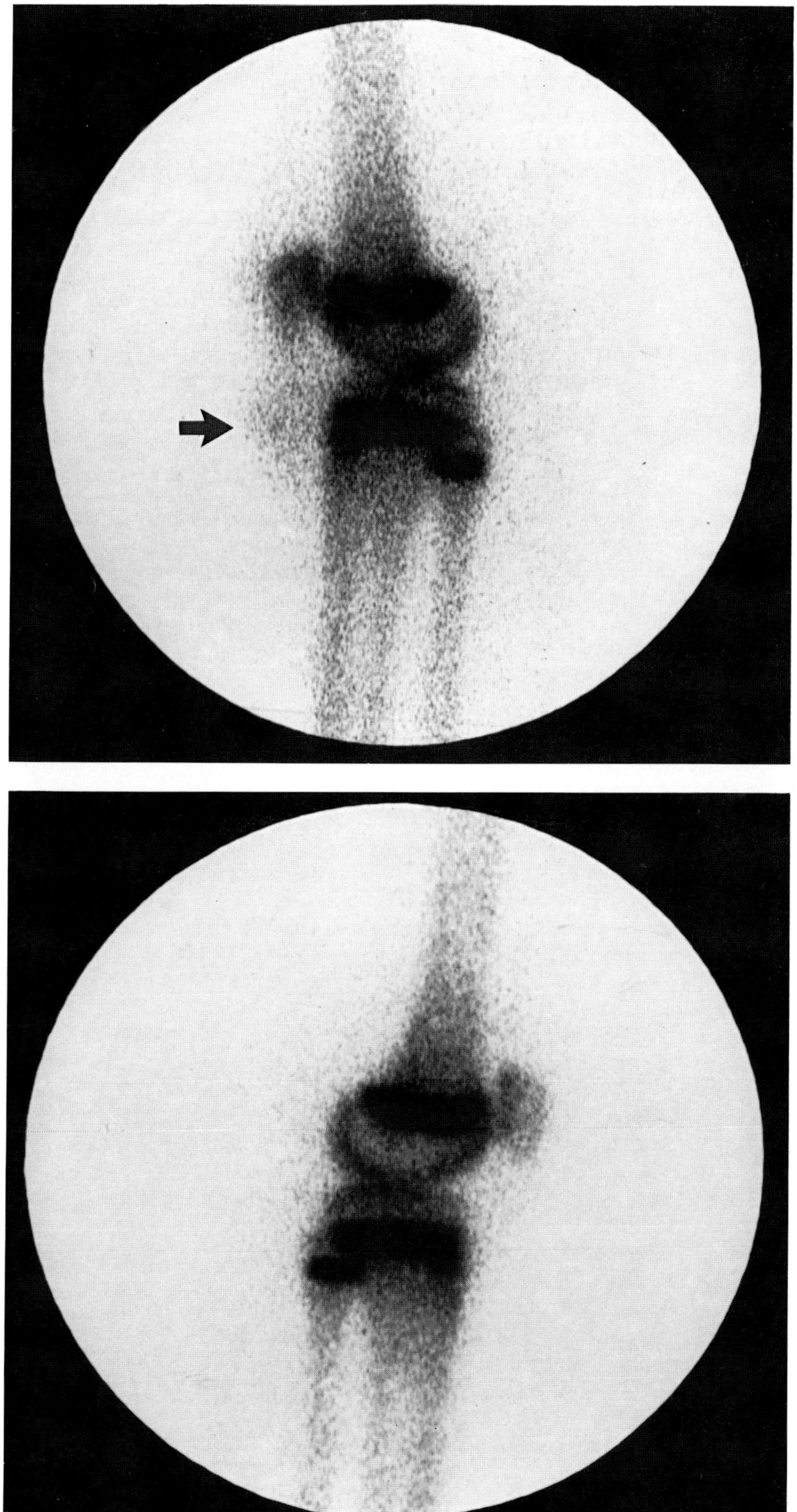

C

D

(Figure 1.20., cont.)

References

1. Matin P. Basic principles of nuclear medicine techniques for detection and evaluation of trauma and sports medicine injuries. *Semin Nucl Med.* 1988; 18:90–112.
2. Francis MD, Fogelman I. ^{99m}Tc diphosphonate uptake mechanisms on bone. In: Fogelman I, ed. *Bone Scanning in Clinical Practice.* London: Springer-Verlag; 1987:7–16.
3. Jung A, Bisaz S, Fleisch H. The binding of pyrophosphate and two diphosphonates by hydroxyapatite crystals. *Calc Tissue Res.* 1973;11:269–280.
4. "S" absorbed dose per unit cumulated activity for selected radionuclides and organs. MIRD Pamphlet No. 11, 1975.
5. Matin P. The appearance of bone scan following fractures including intermediate and long-term studies. *J Nucl Med.* 1979;20:1227–1231.
6. Wahner HW. Radionuclides in the diagnosis of fracture healing. *J Nucl Med.* 1978;19:1356–1358.
7. Gumerman LW, Fogel SR, Goodman MA, et al. Experimental fracture healing: evaluation using radionuclide bone imaging. *J Nucl Med.* 1978;19:1320–1323.
8. Kim HR, Thrall JH, Keyes JW. Skeletal scintigraphy following incidental trauma. *Radiology.* 1979;130:447–451.
9. Medelman JP. Fractures of the sacrum: their incidence in fracture of the pelvis. *Am J Roentgenol.* 1979;42:100.
10. Conolly WB, Hedberg EA. Observations on fractures of the pelvis. *J Trauma.* 1969;9:104.
11. Rosenthall L, Hill RO, Chuang S. Observation on the use of Tc-99m-phosphate imaging in peripheral bone trauma. *Radiology.* 1978;119:637-641.
12. Young MRA, Lowry JH, Ferguson WR. ^{99m}Tc-MDP bone scanning of injuries of the carpal scaphoid. *Injury.* 1988;19:14–17.
13. Ganel A, Engel J, Oster Z, et al. Bone scanning in the assessment of fractures of the scaphoid. *J Hand Surg.* 1979;4:540–453.
14. Rolfe EB, Garvie NW, Khan MA, et al. Isotope bone imaging in suspected scaphoid trauma. *Br J Radiol.* 1981;54:762–767.
15. Dunbar JS, Owen HF, Nogrady MB, et al. Obscure tibial fracture of infants—the toddler's fracture. *J Can Assoc Radiol.* 1964;15:136.
16. Starshak RJ, Simons GW, Stay JR. Occult fracture of the calcaneus—another toddler's fracture. *Pediatr Radiol.* 1984;14:37–40.
17. Clasier CM, Seibert JJ, Williamson SL. The gamut of increased whole bone activity in bone scintigraphy in children. *Clin Nucl Med.* 1987;12:192–197.
18. Borden S. Roentgen recognition of acute plastic bowing of the forearm in children. *Am J Roentgenol.* 1977;125:524–530.
19. Borden S. Traumatic bowing of the forearm in children. *J Bone Joint Surg.* 1974;56A:611–616.
20. Chamay AL. Mechanical and morphological aspects of experimental overload and fatigue in bone. *J Biomech.* 1970;3:263–270.
21. Miller JH, Osterkamp JA. Scintigraphy in acute plastic bowing of the forearm. *Radiology.* 1982;142:742.
22. Zinman H, Keret D, Reis ND. Fracture of the medial sesamoid bone of the hallux. *J Trauma.* 1981;21:581–582.
23. Giannestras NJ, Sammarco GJ. Fractures and dislocations in the foot. In: Rockwood CA, Green DP, eds. *Fractures.* Philadelphia: JB Lippincott Co; 1975:1489–1491.
24. Hohl M, Larson RL. Fractures and dislocations of the knee. In: Rockwood CA, Green DP, eds. *Fractures.* Philadelphia: JB Lippincott Co; 1975:1148–1150.

25. Mandell GA, Alavi A. Scintigraphic evaluation of bone trauma. In: Silberstein T, ed. *Bone Scintigraphy*. Mount Kisco, NY: Futura; 1984:95–144.
26. Pentecost RL, Murray RA, Brindley HH. Fatigue, insufficiency and pathologic fractures. *JAMA*. 1964;187:1001–1004.
27. Zwas ST, Frank G. The role of bone scintigraphy in stress and overuse injuries. In: Freeman LM, Weissman HS, eds. *Nuclear Medicine Annual 1989*. New York: Raven Press; 1989:109–141.
28. Holder LE, Matthews LS. The nuclear physician and sports medicine. In: Freeman LM, Weissman HS, eds. *Nuclear Medicine Annual 1984*. New York: Raven Press; 1984:81–140.
29. Prather JL, Nusynowitz ML, Snowdy HA, et al. Scintigraphic findings in stress fractures. *J Bone Joint Surg*. 1977;59:869–874.
30. Collier BD, Johnson RP, Carrera GF, et al. Painful spondylolysis or spondylolisthesis studied by radiography and single-photon emission computed tomography. *Radiology*. 1985;154:207–211.
31. Mehta RC, Wilson MA. Comparison of planar and SPECT scintigraphy in the detection of spondylolysis. *J Nucl Med*. 1987;28:665. Abstract.
32. Gelfand MJ, Strife JL, Kereiakes JG. Radionuclide bone imaging in spondylolysis of the lumbar spine in children. *Radiology*. 1981;140:191–195.
33. Kleinman PK. Extremity trauma. In: Kleinman PK, ed. *Diagnostic Imaging in Child Abuse*. Baltimore: Williams & Wilkins; 1987:29–66.
34. Jaudes PK. Comparison of radiography and radionuclide bone scanning in the detection of child abuse. *Pediatrics*. 1984;73:166–168.
35. Smith FW, Gilday DL, Ash JM, et al. Unsuspected costovertebral fractures demonstrated by bone scanning in the child abuse syndrome. *Pediatr Radiol*. 1980;10:103–106.
36. Harcke HT. Bone imaging in infants and children: a review. *J Nucl Med*. 1978;19:324–329.
37. Sfakianakis GN, Haase GM, Ortiz VN, et al. The value of bone scanning in early recognition of deliberate child abuse. *J Nucl Med*. 1979;20:675 (abs).
38. Haase GM, Ortiz VN, Sfakianakis GN, et al. The value of radionuclide bone scanning in the early recognition of deliberate child abuse. *J Trauma*. 1980; 20:873–875.
39. Kozin F, Soin JS, Ryan LM, et al. Bone scintigraphy in the reflex sympathetic dystrophy syndrome. *Radiology*. 1981;138:437–443.
40. Kozin F. The painful shoulder and the reflex sympathetic dystrophy syndrome. In: McCarty DJ, ed. *Arthritis and Allied Conditions*. Philadelphia: Lea & Febiger; 1979:1091–1120.
41. Vogler JB III, Genant HK. Osteoporosis. In: Taveras JM, Ferucci JT, eds. *Radiology*. Philadelphia: JB Lippincott Co; 1986:5;12.
42. Arnstein A. Regional osteoporosis. *Ortho Clin North Am*. 1972;3:585–600.
43. Rosen PS, Graham W. The shoulder-hand syndrome: historical review with observations on seventy-three patients. *Can Med Assoc J*. 1957;77:86–91.
44. Demangeat JL, Constantinesco A, Brunot B, et al. Three-phase bone scanning in reflex sympathetic dystrophy of the hand. *J Nucl Med*. 1988;29:26–32.
45. Feldman N, Heyman S. Skeletal scintigraphic findings in children with reflex sympathetic dystrophy. *J Nucl Med*. 1986;27:932. Abstract
46. Matin P. Bone scintigraphy in the diagnosis and management of traumatic injury. *Semin Nucl Med*. 1983;13:104–122.
47. Forsted DL, Dalinka MK, Mitchell E, et al. Radiologic evaluation of treatment of nonunion of fractures by electrical stimulation. *Radiology*. 1978; 128:629–634.
48. U.S. Public Health Service Vital and Health Statistics Series, National Health Survey, Series 10. 1967;57:30.
49. Desai A, Alavi A, Dalinka M, et al. Role of scintigraphy in the evaluation

and treatment of nonunited fractures: concise communication. *J Nucl Med.* 1980;21:931–934.
50. Alavi A, Desai A, Esterhai J, et al. Bone scanning in the evaluation of nonunited fractures. *J Nucl Med.* 1979;20:647. Abstract
51. Rosenthall L, Lisbona R. Role of radionuclide imaging in benign bone and joint disease of orthopedic interest. In: Freeman LM, Weissman HS, eds. *Nuclear Medicine Annual 1980.* New York: Raven Press; 1980.
52. Riggins RL, DeNardo GL, D'Ambrosia R, et al. Assessment of circulation in the femoral head by fluorine-18 scintigraphy. *J Nucl Med.* 1974;15:183–186.
53. Morley TR, Short MD, Dorsett DJ. Femoral head activity in Perthes' disease: Clinical evaluation of quantitative technique for estimating tracer uptake. *J Nucl Med.* 1978;19:884–901.
54. Ogden JA, Southwick WO: Osgood-Schlatter's disease and tibial tuberosity development. *Clin Orthop.* 1976;116:180–188.

CHAPTER 2

Atlas of SPECT Cross-Sectional Anatomy of the Normal Spine, Pelvis, Hips, and Skull

Gary F. Gates, Dov Front, Harvey Ziessman, and Ora Israel

The radionuclide bone scan is one of the most commonly performed examinations in nuclear medicine departments worldwide. This procedure has been improved continually over the past several decades by advances in both radiopharmaceuticals and imaging equipment. Currently, bone scanning is generally regarded as one of the most sensitive imaging studies available for detecting focal osseous abnormalities, and with the development of single photon emission computed tomography (SPECT), further refinement has been experienced. However, SPECT requires more attention to details of acquisition, processing, and interpretation. Detailed technical discussions of bone SPECT acquisition and processing have been the subjects of other publications and will not be covered here. This chapter is devoted to normal SPECT skeletal anatomy.

In general, interpretation of all imaging examinations can be conceived as occurring in three stages: a) recognition of an abnormality, b) anatomic localization of the abnormality, and c) diagnosis of the etiology of the abnormality. However, unfamiliarity with basic anatomy or failure to recognize normal structures in the images may result in incorrect interpretations. This is especially important with SPECT skeletal imaging. Improved lesion detection with precision in anatomic localization is justification for SPECT bone scanning. The improvement in lesion detection is due to increased contrast enhancement as well as elimination, due to the tomographic effect, of adjacent overlapping structures that may obscure an area. Precision in anatomic localization of an abnormal site of tracer uptake is a consequence of the tomographic process, an important aspect of diagnostic accuracy.

This chapter is concerned with normal anatomy of the thoracic spine, lumbosacral spine, pelvis, hips, and skull. The superiority of SPECT bone imaging over planar studies has been documented, and once having used this procedure, most practitioners of clinical nuclear medicine soon come to realize the advantages of SPECT imaging. A practical consequence of this improved scintigraphic technique is a more meaningful consultation with referring physicians and diagnostic radiologists regarding which specific anatomic region should be evaluated further by other imaging examinations. It is no longer adequate when discussing a scan with these colleagues, to refer to a vertebra as being "abnormal." They want to know exactly where the lesion is located (i.e., vertebral body, lamina, spinous process, etc.). The rest of this chapter is devoted to SPECT anatomy of the regions mentioned in order that one may recognize normal structures and correctly localize focal lesions. Further reading is available.[1–9]

Gross Anatomy of the Spine

Thoracic and Lumbar Vertebrae

The vertebral column is composed of 24 true vertebrae (7 cervical, 12 thoracic, 5 lumbar) plus two composite vertebrae (sacrum and coccyx) and has a complex series of compensating curves. Those portions of the spine located posterior to bony cavities have a concave anterior curvature (i.e., thoracic spine behind thoracic cage; sacrum and coccyx behind bony pelvis) whereas the cervical and lumbar spines have a convex anterior curvature in compensation. Specific morphological details of the thoracic and lumbar spine plus sacrum and coccyx need to be addressed in order to analyze these regions using bone SPECT imaging.

The descriptive terminology regarding joints needs to be briefly mentioned. There are three general classifications of joints: a) synarthroses (immovable, such as skull sutures), b) amphiarthroses (slightly mobile, such as between vertebral bodies with "symphysis" being the name given to the subclassification in this example), and c) diarthroses (freely moveable, with subclassification "arthrodia" describing the gliding motion between articular processes of vertebrae).

In general, a vertebra is composed of two parts: a body and a vertebral (neural) arch. The anterior segment (body) provides weight support while the posterior component (vertebral arch) encloses the vertebral foramen through which the spinal cord passes. Lumbar vertebral bodies have a greater transverse diameter than anteroposterior, whereas these dimensions are relatively equal in thoracic vertebrae.

The cylindrical-shaped vertebral bodies are separated from each other by the intervertebral disks. These structures are attached to the thin layers of hyaline cartilage covering the opposing surfaces of contiguous vertebrae. These fibrocartilaginous structures, which also attach to the anterior longitudinal ligament in front and posterior longitudinal ligament behind, serve as the principal connecting elements between vertebrae. These slightly mobile joints created by the intervertebral disks are classified as amphiarthroses subclassification "symphysis." The anterior longitudinal ligament is attached to fibrocartilaginous disks as well as adjacent margins of the vertebrae; this thick, broad band contacts the middle part of the body but is not attached to it. The posterior longitudinal ligament is also attached to the disks and contiguous vertebral margins, but this narrow, thick band is separated from the surface of the middle part of the body by the basivertebral veins. This latter situation has been offered as a partial explanation for the posterior direction of herniated disks or their fragments. The intervertebral disks account for about 25% of the length of the vertebral column but this percentage is not uniformly distributed throughout since the cervical and lumbar regions have thicker disks, relative to vertebral body length, than the thoracic area. This allows for greater motion in cervical and lumbar areas compared to the thoracic region. The disks function as shock absorbers for vertically directed forces (i.e., cranial to caudal or vice versa).

The vertebral arch is a more complex structure than the body and is composed of two pedicles, two laminae, and seven processes. The processes are classified as articular (four), transverse (two), and spinous (one).

The pedicles are short, thick, bony structures extending posteriorly from the upper and posterolateral surfaces of the vertebral foramen and form a bridge from the vertebral body to the lamina. Concavities along the superior and inferior vertebral margins of the pedicles are identified as the superior and inferior vertebral notches, respectively. The superior notch is smaller than the inferior notch. Adjacent superior and inferior notches of articulating vertebrae form intervertebral foramen through which spinal nerves and vessels pass.

The laminae are broad plates extending medially and posteriorly from the pedicles. They fuse in the midline and form the posterior boundary of the vertebral foramen. The anterior margin of the vertebral foramen is formed by the posterior surface of the vertebrae whereas the pedicles comprise the lateral margins. A vertebral foramen in the lumbar area is triangular whereas a thoracic foramina tend to be circular. The lamina of the thoracic spine are imbricated (i.e., each overlapping the next lowermost lamina like tiles or shingles on a roof). Lumbar lamina do not overlap each other.

The spinous process has its base at the midline junction of laminae and is directed posteriorly. Thoracic spinous processes are also angled sharply downward, especially in the midthoracic region, whereas this angulation is less prominent in the very low thoracic and lumbar regions. Thoracic spinous processes are more spike-shaped compared to lumbar processes, which are larger and more oblong.

The four articular processes arise at the junction of pedicles with the lamina. Two articular processes extend upward (superior articular processes) whereas the remaining two are directed downward (inferior articular processes). Thoracic superior processes have their articular surface directed posteriorly whereas the articular surface of the lumbar superior processes have a posterior and medial contour. Inferior processes of the thoracic spine have their articular surfaces directed anteriorly but these surfaces on processes in the lumbar region have an anterior and lateral orientation. The articular processes come into apposition with the corresponding processes of adjacent vertebrae above and below. The articulating surface of each process is called a facet, and a pair of facets form an apophyseal joint. The gliding joints formed between the articular facets are classified as arthrodial (subclassification of diarthroses) and comprise an articular capsule attached to the margins of adjacent articular processes. These capsules are lined by synovial membranes forming a cavity filled with synovial fluid. These joints restrict motion in some directions while allowing it in others and are especially important in preventing forward slippage of the vertebral bodies. Defects (either developmental or after trauma) within both interarticular portions of the lamina (pars interarticularis) result in a separation of the vertebra into two components: a) an anterior portion consisting of a vertebral body attached to pedicles, transverse processes, and superior articular processes, and b) a posterior segment consisting of inferior articular processes connected to lamina and spinous process. This is termed spondylolysis, which over time may allow for forward displacement of the vertebral body (spondylolisthesis). The superior articular processes are still in contact with the inferior ones from the adjacent vertebra above but the lack of connection with the inferior articular processes is destabilizing and produces a hinge effect superiorly (through the superior processes), resulting in anterior displacement of the inferior surface of the vertebral body. A unilateral pars interarticularis defect is usually unassociated with spondylolisthesis.

Transverse processes project laterally from the vertebral arch and generally arise near the junction of the laminae with the pedicles; they are located between superior and inferior articular processes. Regional variations occur. Thoracic transverse processes arise from the lamina portion of the vertebral arch behind the pedicles and superior articular processes. Upper lumbar transverse processes (L1-3) arise at the junction of the pedicles and laminae whereas those at L4-5 originate further forward near the intersection of the pedicles and posterior portions of the vertebrae bodies. Lumbar transverse processes are in front of the articular processes contrasted to their thoracic counterparts, which are located behind the articular processes. Lumbar transverse processes are long, slender and point laterally whereas thoracic ones are relatively thicker and are directed posteriorly, laterally, and upward. The transverse processes of the thoracic spine are longest in the upper portions of the spine and gradually shorten as the lower regions are approached. The first through tenth ribs articulate with vertebrae as well as transverse processes. The rib tubercles articulate with a facet located along the anterior tip of the transverse processes (costotransverse joints) whereas rib heads articulate along the posterior and lateral vertebral body surfaces by means of a series of facets and demifacets (costocentral or costovertebral joints). Ribs 11 and 12 articulate only with vertebral bodies and not with transverse processes. The heads of ribs 1, 10, 11, and 12 articulate solely with a facet at their corresponding vertebral body. However, ribs 2 through 9 articulate with two demifacets located near the superior and inferior vertebral body margins and with the interposed intervertebral fibrocartilages; the combination of two demifacets and disk margin serves as a functional joint. The costotransverse and costovertebral joints are arthrodial or gliding joints surrounded by an articular capsule and lined by a synovial membrane.

Sacral and Coccygeal Vertebrae

The sacrum comprises five segments, and the coccyx generally comprises four. These segments unite forming the sacrum and coccyx of adulthood, and thus they are composite vertebrae.

The triangular sacrum is positioned like a wedge separating the ilia of the pelvis. The base articulates with the lowermost lumbar vertebra and projects forward forming the lumbosacral or sacrovertebral angle (measured as Ferguson's normal lumbosacral angle of 34°). The central portion of the sacrum is projected backwards with a concave anterior curvature. The lower most portion, or apex, angles forward and articulates with the coccyx. Broad bony processes (sacral ala) extend out laterally from the central vertebral bodies producing a winged appearance; their lateral margins articulate with the inner margins of the ilia forming the sacroiliac joints. A vertebral canal, triangular in shape above, runs the length of the sacrum and harbors sacral nerves that exit via four pairs of anterior and posterior sacral foramina on each side. The lower posterior wall of the vertebral canal may be incomplete owing to poorly developed laminae and spinous processes. An intervertebral disk is located at the junction of the lowermost lumbar vertebra and superior surface of the first sacral vertebra forming an amphiarthrodial joint. The sacroiliac articulation is also an amphiarthrodial joint; cartilaginous plates cover the two articular surfaces and are interconnected to some degree by softer fibrocartilage and interosseous fibers superiorly and inferiorly. A small space containing synovial-like fluid separates the joint components and thus these have some features of diarthrosis. Anterior and posterior sacroiliac ligaments plus interosseous ligaments cover the joint.

The fused segments forming the coccyx lack pedicles, laminae, and spinous processes. This small bony appendage articulating with the apex of the sacrum is directed anteriorly and downward. The sacrococcygeal joint or symphysis is an amphiarthrodial joint.

Gross Anatomy of the Pelvis, Hip, and Femoral Head

The pelvis comprises three bones: the ilium, ischium, and pubis. The pelvis has three joints including one symphysis pubis and two sacroiliac joints.

The ilium is fan-shaped and concave. The upper aspect is the iliac crest, which extends from the posterior superior iliac spine sinuously to the anterior superior iliac spine. The anterior aspect of the ilium joins with the ischium and pubis to form the cup-shaped acetabulum for the head of the femur. Posteriorly, the ilium articulates with the ala of the sacrum at the sacroiliac joints. The ischium has three parts including a body, a tuberosity, and a ramus. The body of the ischium is triangular and joins the ilium. The tuberosity is an enlarged ovoid bony area, which projects downward from the body and forms the ischial tuberosity. The ischial ramus extends forward and superiorly to the inferior public ramus. The pubis has three parts including a body, a superior ramus, and an inferior ramus. The body of the pubis articulates with its counterpart from the opposite side forming the symphysis pubis. The superior ramus extends laterally from the body and fuses with the ilium to form part of the acetabulum. The inferior ramus extends laterally from the body of the pubis and joins with the ramus of the ischium.

The proximal portion of the femur is formed by the head, neck, greater trochanter, and lesser trochanter. The head has a spherical shape and extends medial and superiorly into the acetabulum. The neck extends laterally and inferiorly from the head. The lesser trochanter is a result of the traction on the epiphysis by the iliopsoas muscle. It extends medially from the posterior surface of the femur. The greater trochanter is a result of the traction on the epiphysis by the gluteus medius and the gluteus minimus. It extends superiorly, posteriorly, and medially.

Gross Anatomy of the Skull

The gross anatomy of the bones of the skull is complex, and an in-depth discussion is beyond the scope of this atlas. The reader is referred to the many excellent atlases of gross anatomy. This section discusses the gross anatomy of the bones of the skull, which can be identified in SPECT images, and these are identified on the various coronal, transverse, and sagittal SPECT images that follow. As SPECT also improves, a more in-depth understanding of the gross anatomy of the bones of the skull will be required.

Atlas Section

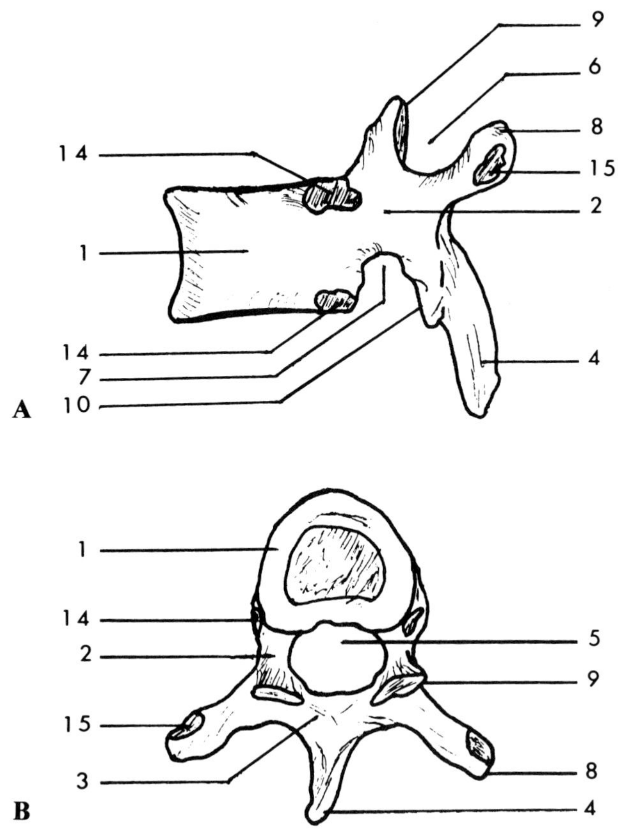

The Thoracic and Lumbosacral Area

Figure 2.1. Thoracic vertebra – schematic.

This line drawing depicts a midthoracic vertebra as viewed from the left side (**A**) and from the top (**B**).

Numerical code to thoracic and lumbosacral images (figures 2.1–2.11):

1. Vertebral body
2. Pedicle
3. Lamina
4. Spinous process
5. Vertebral foramen
6. Superior vertebral notch
7. Inferior vertebral notch
8. Transverse process
9. Superior articular process
10. Inferior articular process
11. Intervertebral disk space
12. Intervertebral foramen
13. Pars interarticularis region
14. Demifacet for costovertebral joint
15. Facet for costotransverse joint
16. Sacral body
17. Sacral ala
18. Coccyx
19. Costovertebral or costotransverse joint
20. Rib
21. Scapula
22. Sternum
23. Sacroiliac joint
24. Ilium
25. Facet Joint

Figure 2.2. Lumbar vertebra—schematic.

This line drawing depicts a midlumbar vertebra as viewed from the left side (**A**) and from the top (**B**). (Numerical codes are found in the caption of Figure 2.1.)

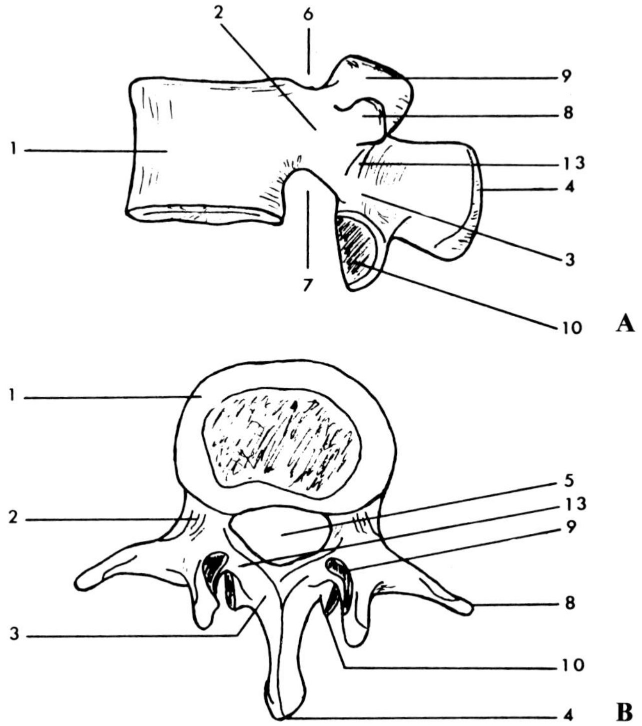

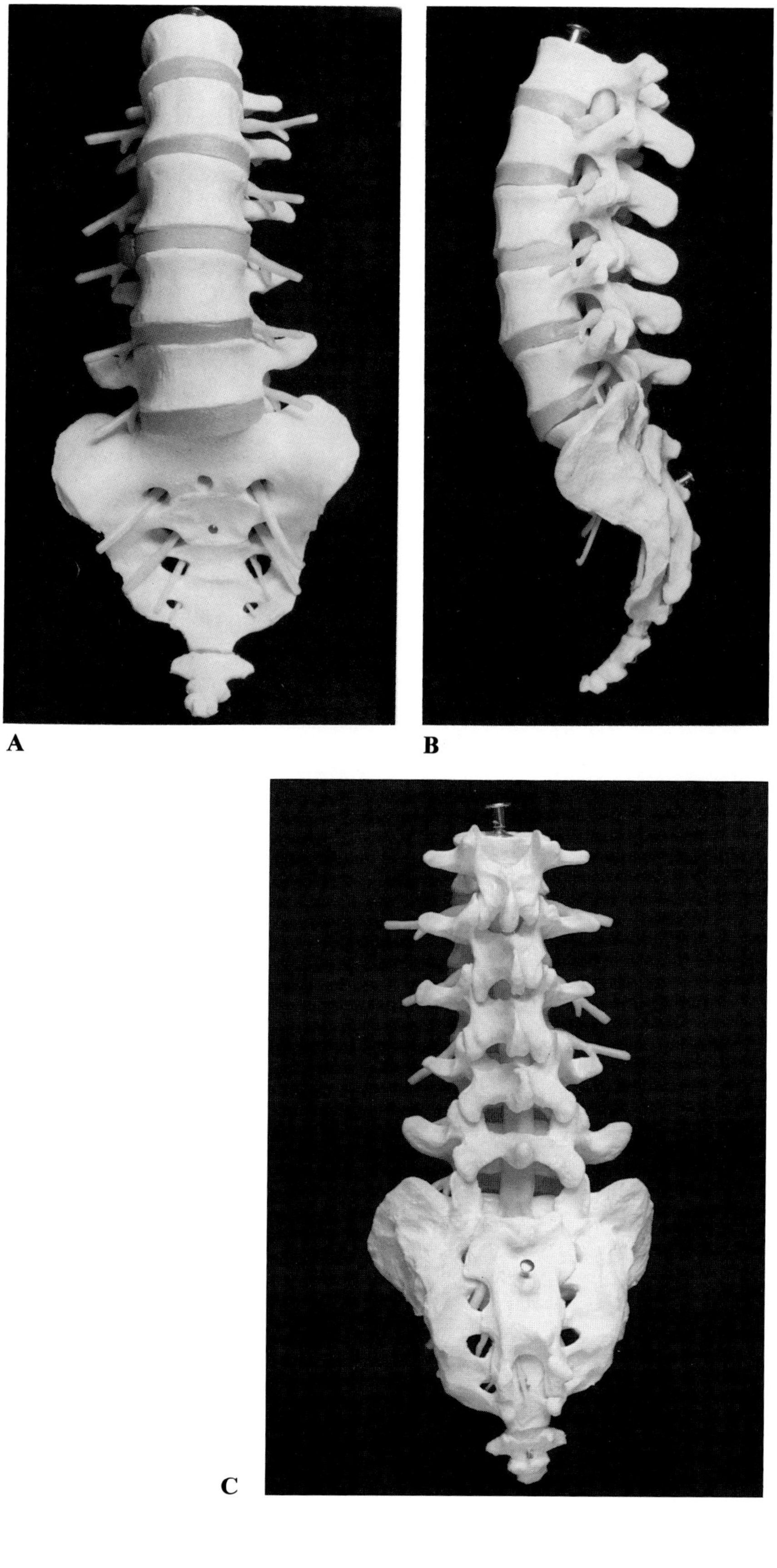

A B C

Figure 2.3. Model of lumbar spine.

This model of the lumbar spine illustrates the relationship of the vertebrae (**A–C**).

Figure 2.4. Thoracic spine (coronal).

A–D: Serial coronal sections of the thoracic spine from anterior to posterior.
Comment: The anterior concavity of the thoracic spine varies from patient to patient and tends to increase with age owing to the gradual development of a kyphotic curvature. As a result, the lower thoracic vertebral bodies are visualized before upper ones. The vertebral bodies are readily identifiable, but the disc spaces are not as easily demonstrated as in the lumbar region. Likewise, the spinous processes are not as well visualized as in the lumbar spine, because they are downwardly directed and overlapping. The ribs articulate with the vertebrae in a complex manner. The heads of all ribs articulate with vertebral bodies by either a facet or two demifacets (costovertebral joints), and ribs 1 through 10 also articulate with transverse processes (costotransverse joints). The articular points of the transverse processes with the posterior, medial components of the curved ribs are close to the apophyseal joints formed by the facets on the superior and inferior articular processes of the vertebrae. The close proximity of these sites (in combination with the relatively more prominent transverse processes in the upper thoracic spine) not only results in a widened appearance of the upper and midthoracic spine but also makes it difficult to distinguish between the apophyseal joint area, costotransvérse joints, and especially costovertebral joint regions. The above is further demonstrated in Figs. 2.5 and 2.6. The thoracic vertebrae 11 and 12 have only costovertebral joints. (Numerical codes are found in the caption of Figure 2.1.)

Figure 2.4. continued on following page

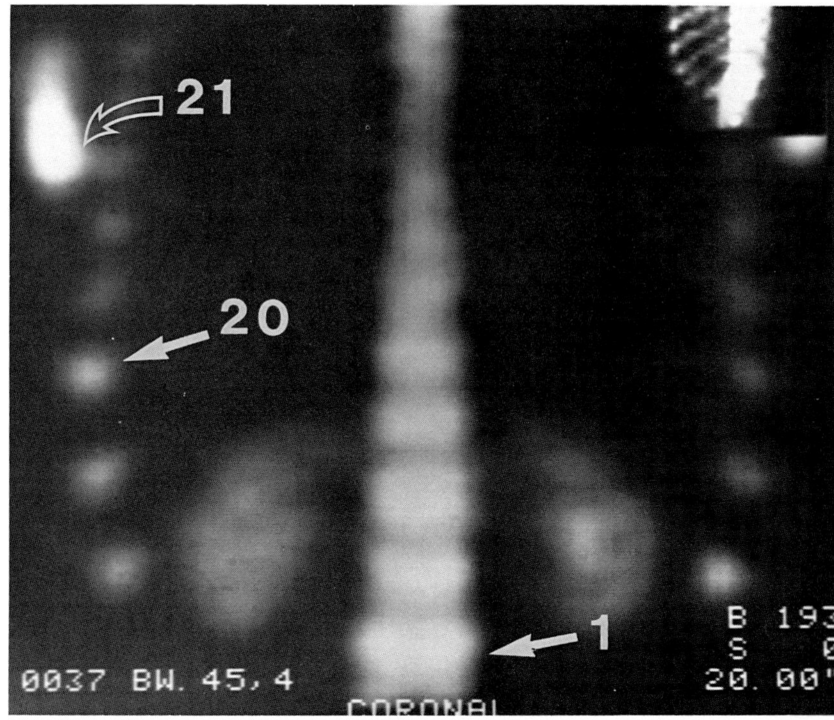

A

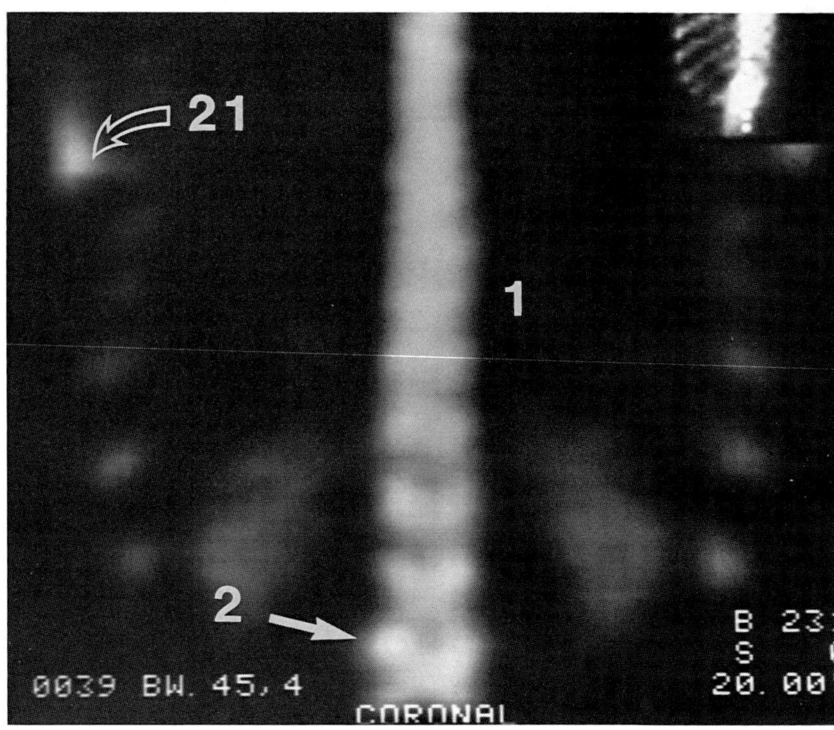

B

(Figure 2.4., cont.)

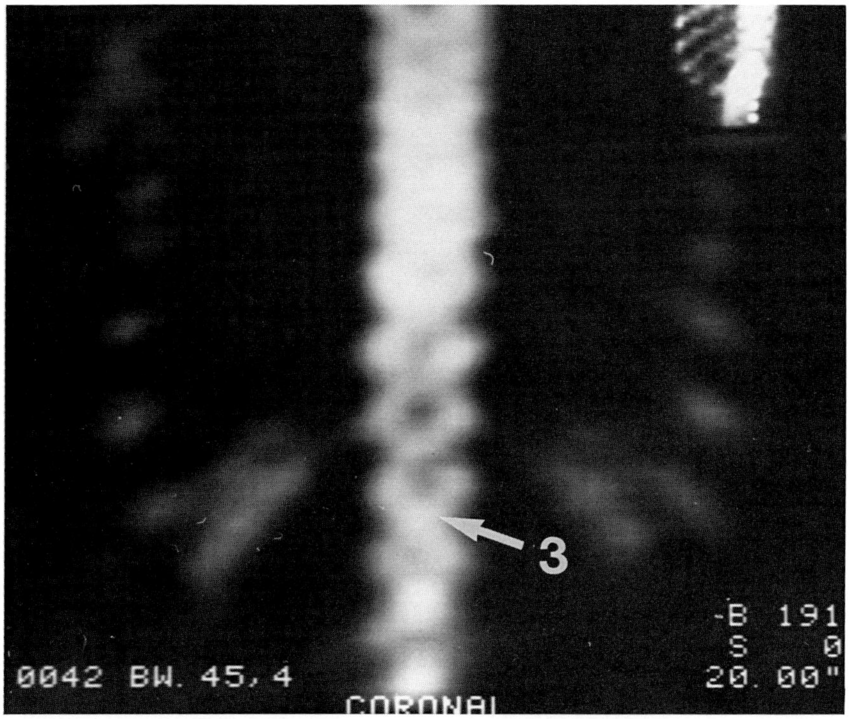

C

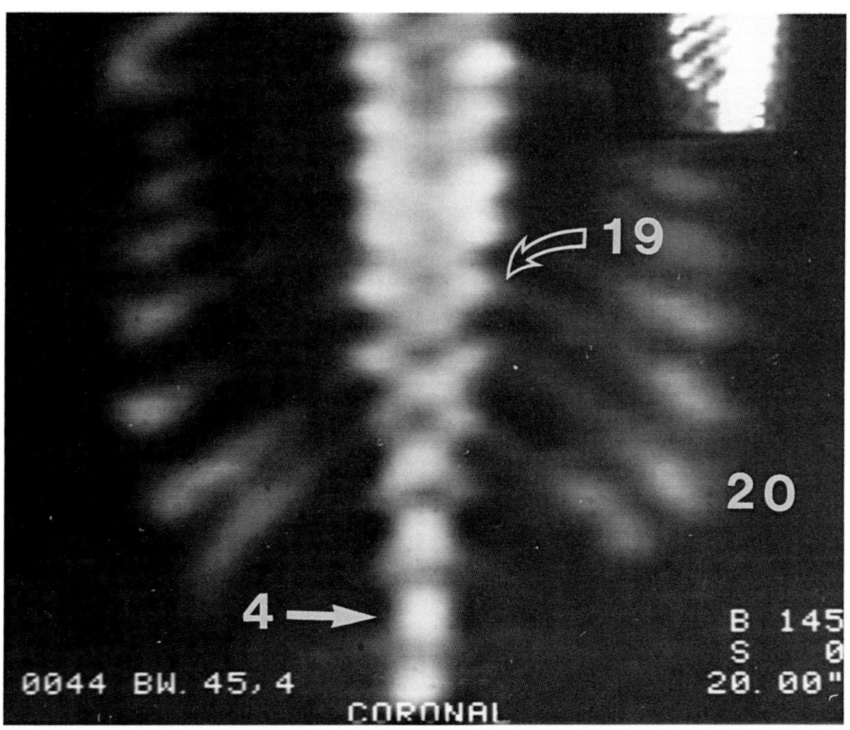

D

Figure 2.5. Thoracic spine (sagittal).

This midline sagittal section shows the linear arrangement of vertebrae from the upper thoracic to lumbar areas.
Comment: Sagittal sections show all the vertebrae on one film with the midsagittal view displaying the vertebral bodies best. As discussed previously, the spinous processes of the thoracic vertebrae are not as well visualized as in the lumbar spine, because they are downwardly directed and overlapping. Likewise, the intervertebral disc spaces in the lumbar area show more clearly than in the thoracic region. The sternum is seen anterior to the thoracic spine. (Numerical codes are found in the caption of Figure 2.1.)

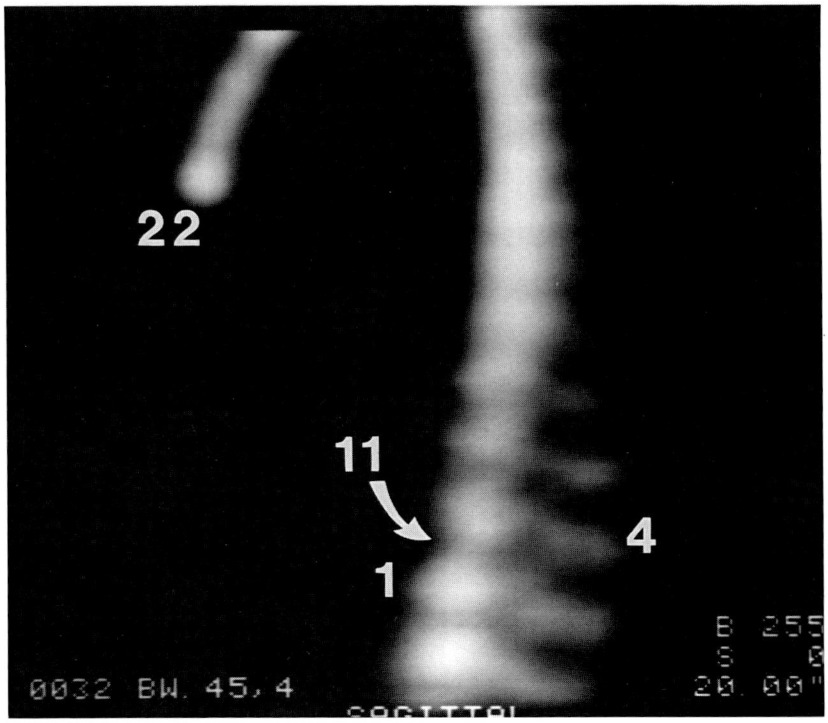

Figure 2.6. Thoracic spine (transverse) with demonstration of costovertebral and costotransverse joints.

These transverse sections are at the level of T-11 (**A** and **B**) and T-10 (**C** and **D**). Different photographic intensities were used to illustrate the vertebral bodies, vertebral foramen, and articulations with the ribs. **E** demonstrates the costotransverse joint well.
Comments: Transverse sections show vertebral body, foramen, and arch on one view. Careful formatting can also pick up the rib articulations. Notice that in the region of the posterior elements, T-11 has a more narrow appearance as compared to T-10; T-10 has a costotransverse articulation where as T-11 and T-12 do not. The transverse processes with costotransverse articulations are more prominent in the up-

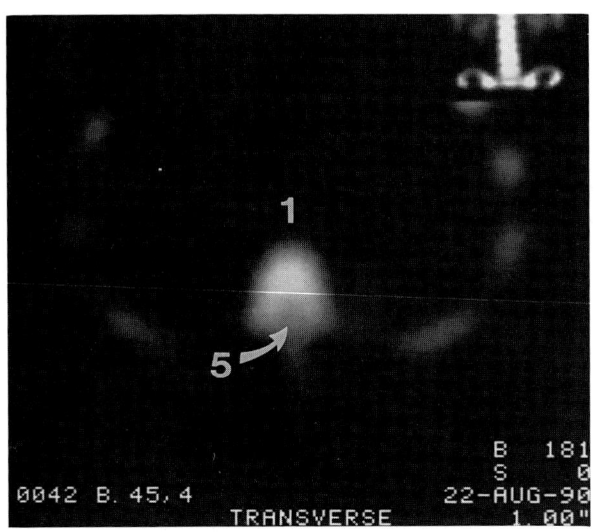

A

Figure 2.6. continued on following page

(Figure 2.6., cont.)

per rather than lower spine, which results in the configuration of a narrow isosceles triangle on coronal sections (see Fig. 2.4D) (base superior and apex pointed down). Some transverse sections demonstrate the costotransverse joints along with other features of the vertebral anatomy **(E)** especially well. (Numerical codes are found in the caption of Figure 2.1.)

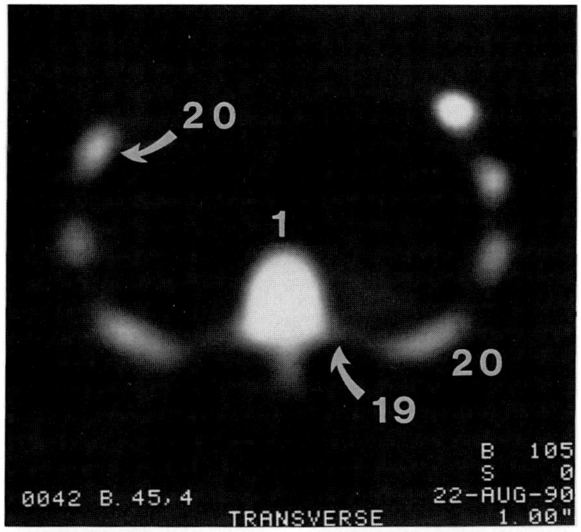

B

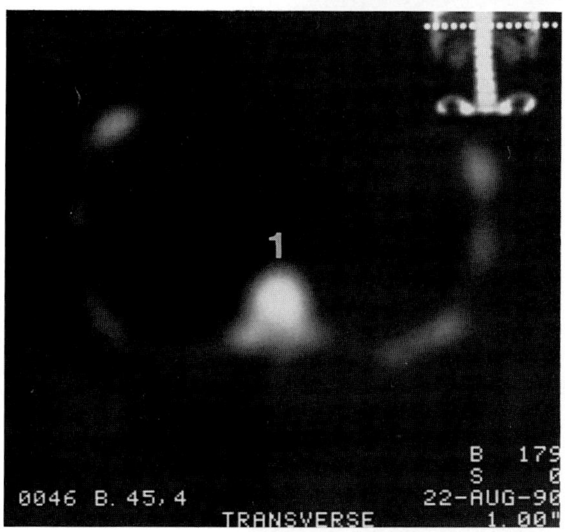

C

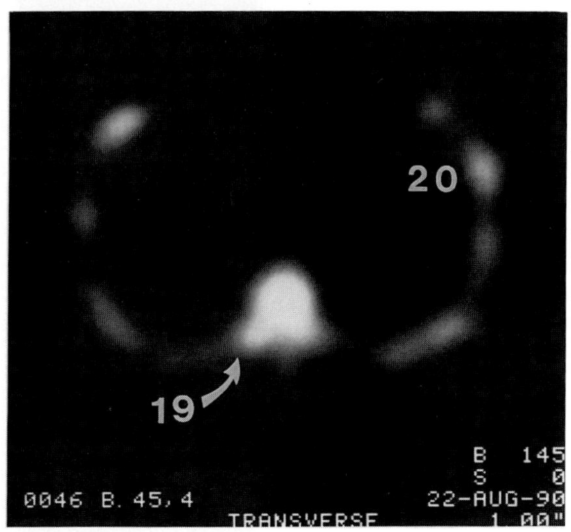

D

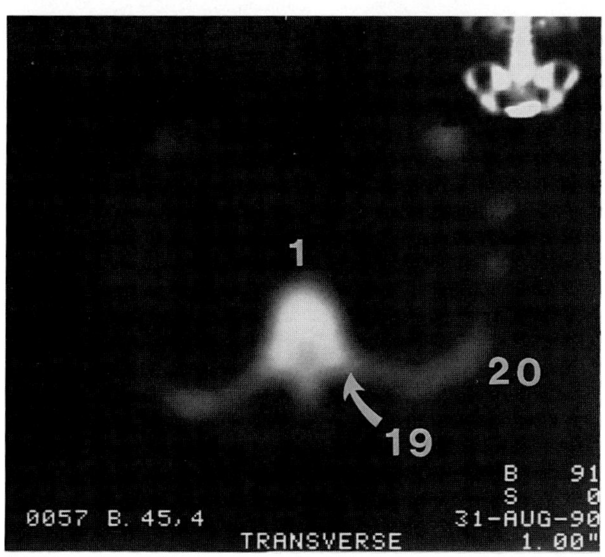

E

Figure 2.7. Thoracic spine (coronal) with demonstration of costovertebral and costotransverse joints.

These serial anterior to posterior images (**A–E**) show the configuration of the thoracic spine at the level of the rib articulations.

Comments: The most posterior sections give a sense of rib curvature especially in the uppermost portions of the thoracic region. Notice how the spinous processes ultimately appear as a linear arrangement of focal points. (Numerical codes are found in the caption of Figure 2.1.)

Figure 2.7. continued on following page

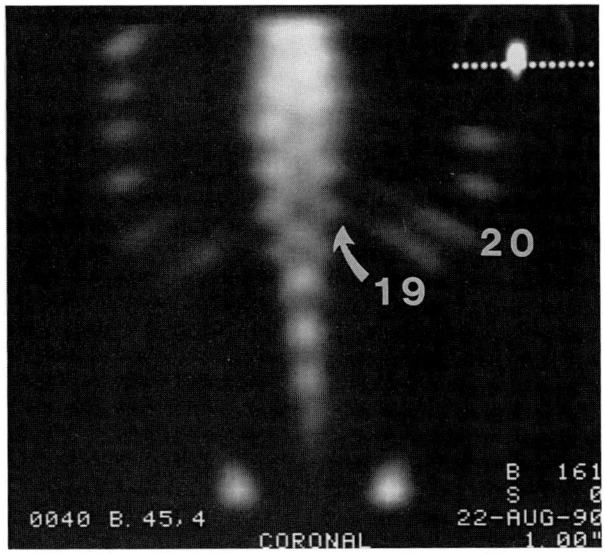

A

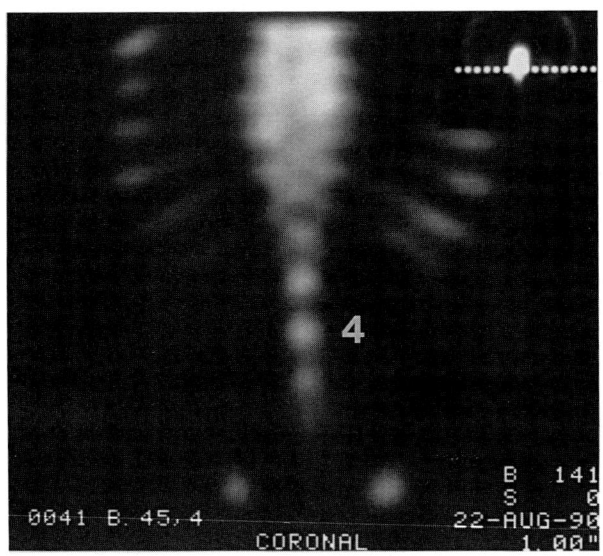

B

(Figure 2.7., cont.)

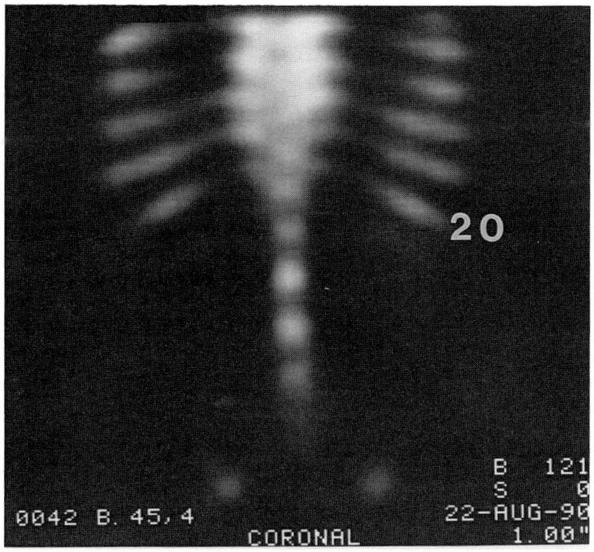

C

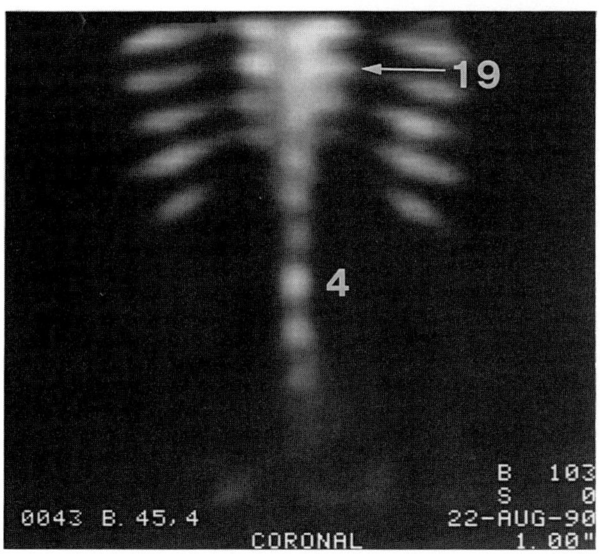

D

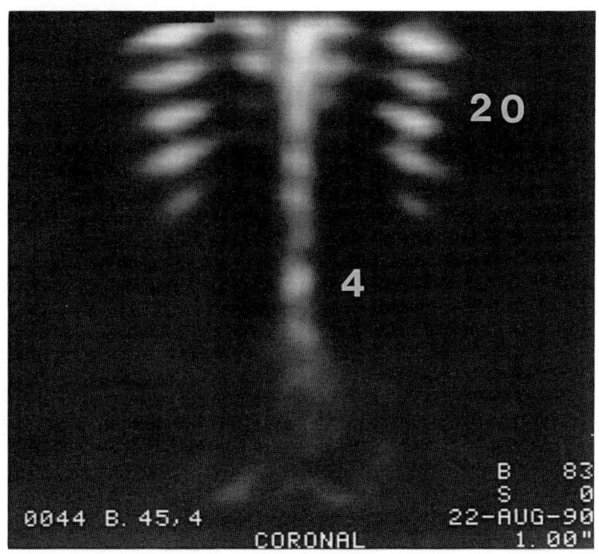

E

Figure 2.8. Ribs (sagittal).

A, which is a sagittal section in the lateral aspect of the thorax, demonstrates the linear appearance of ribs, which should be compared to the appearance of the ribs in a more medial sagittal section (**B**). In the latter, the ribs have an anterior and posterior segmental appearance. The scapula is also seen. (Numerical codes are found in the caption of Figure 2.1.)

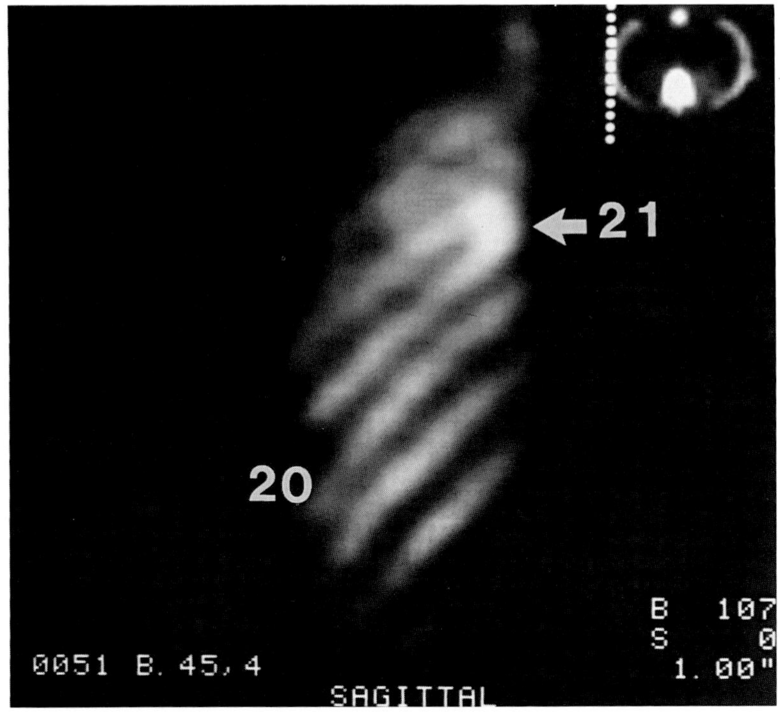

A

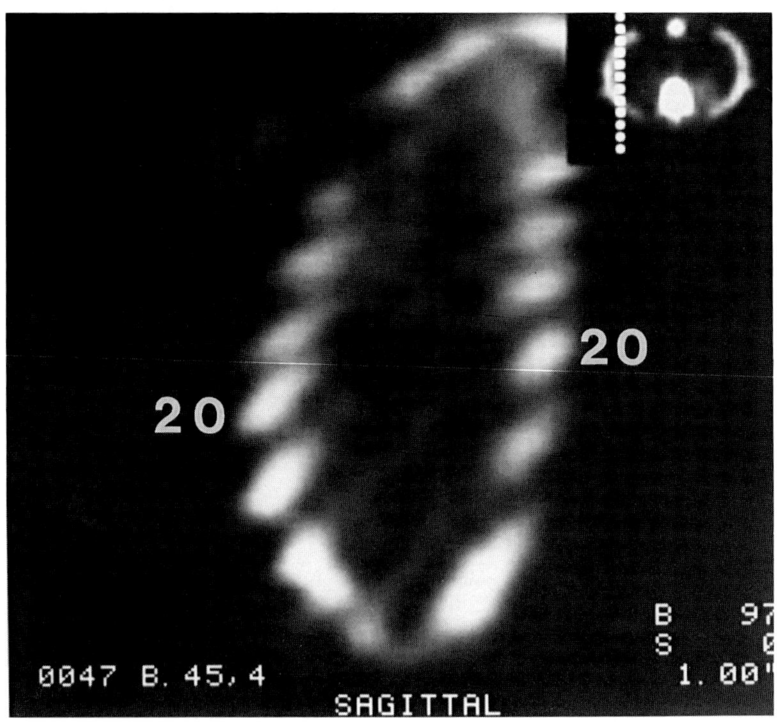

B

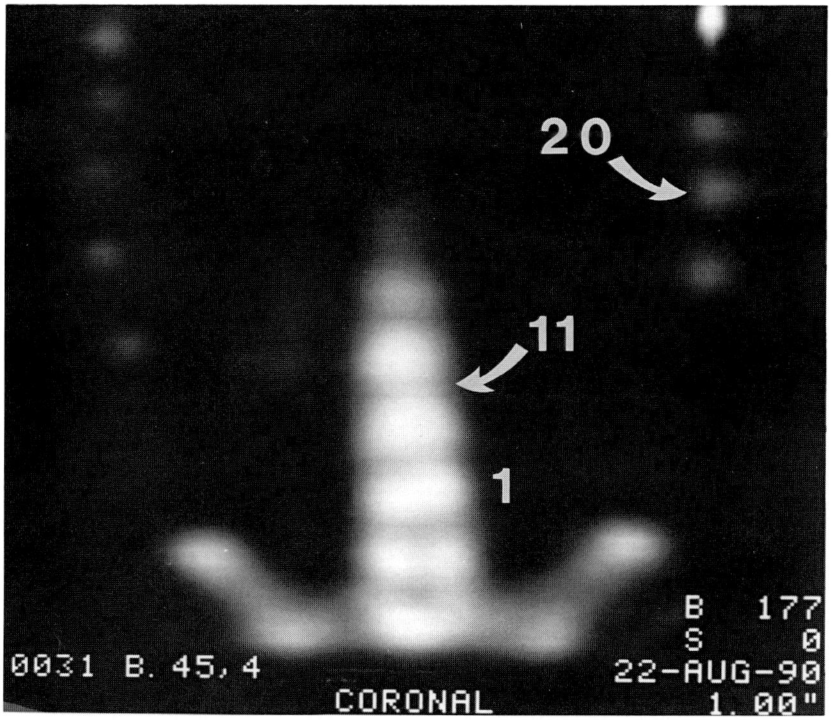

A

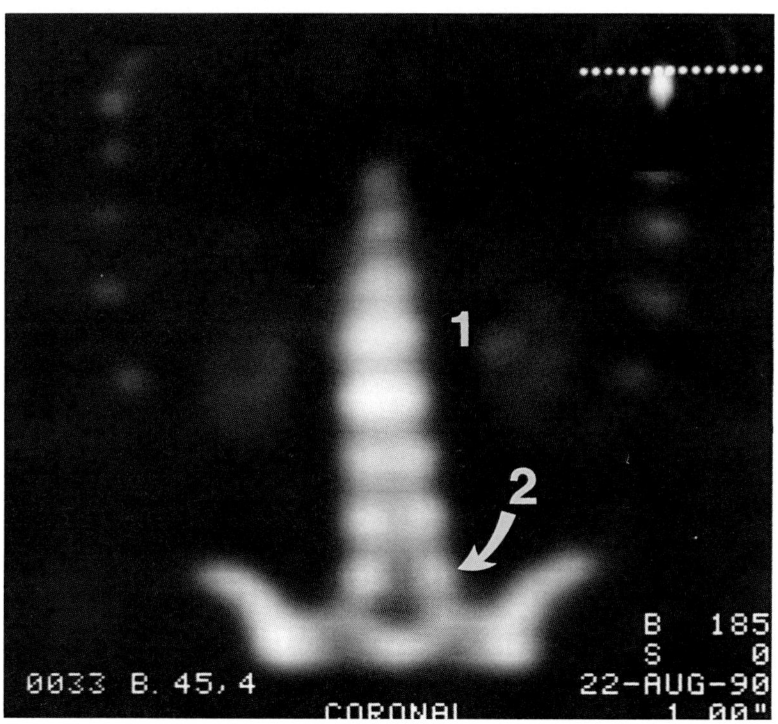

B

Figure 2.9. Thoracolumbar spine (coronal and sagittal).

Serial anterior to posterior coronal sections (**A–F**) show a smooth and sequential appearance of the lumbar and lower thoracic vertebrae. Midline sagittal view (**G**) shows the variable appearance of thoracic versus lumbar spinous processes whereas a more lateral, parasagittal section (**H**) shows the pedicles and intervertebral foramen. (Numerical codes are found in the caption of Figure 2.1.)

Figure 2.9. continued on following pages

(Figure 2.9., cont.)

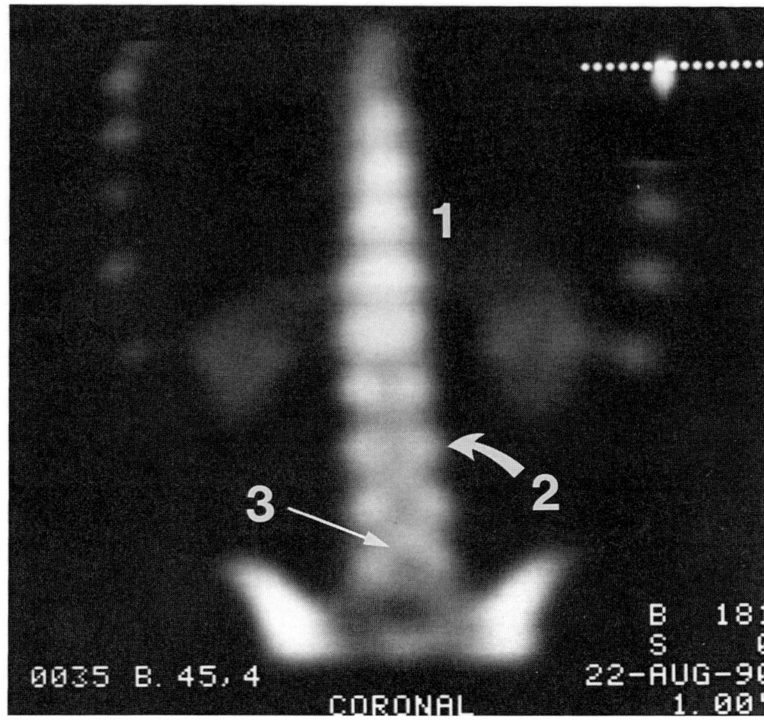

C

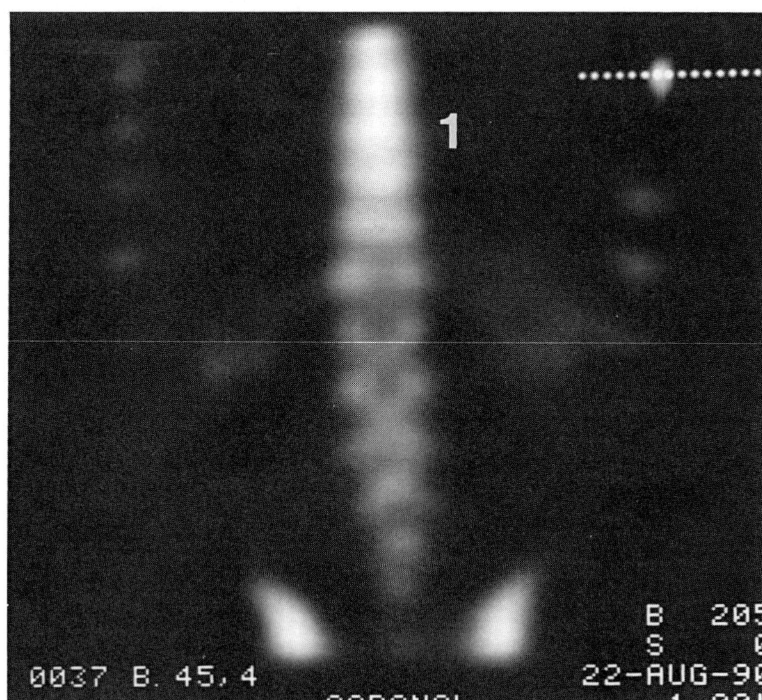

D

(Figure 2.9., cont.)

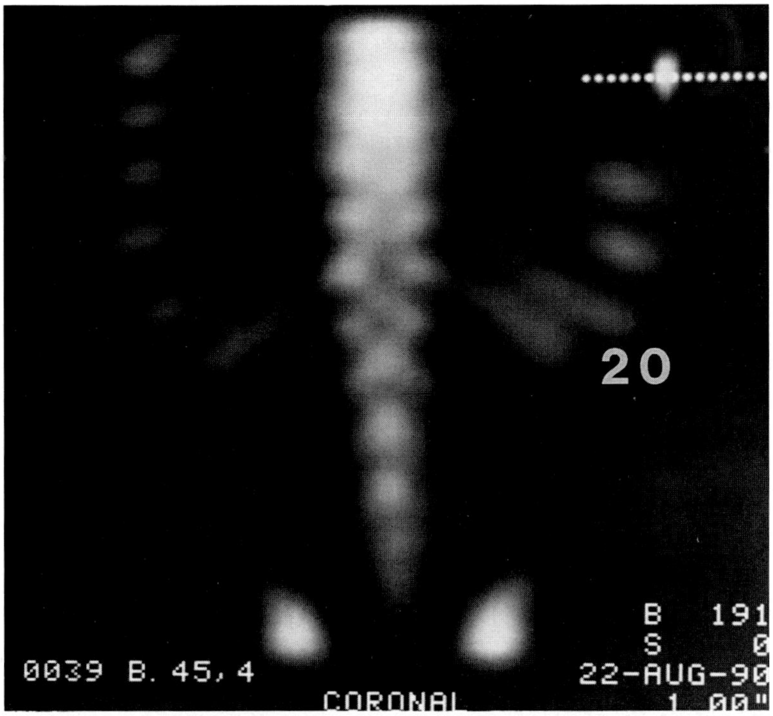

E

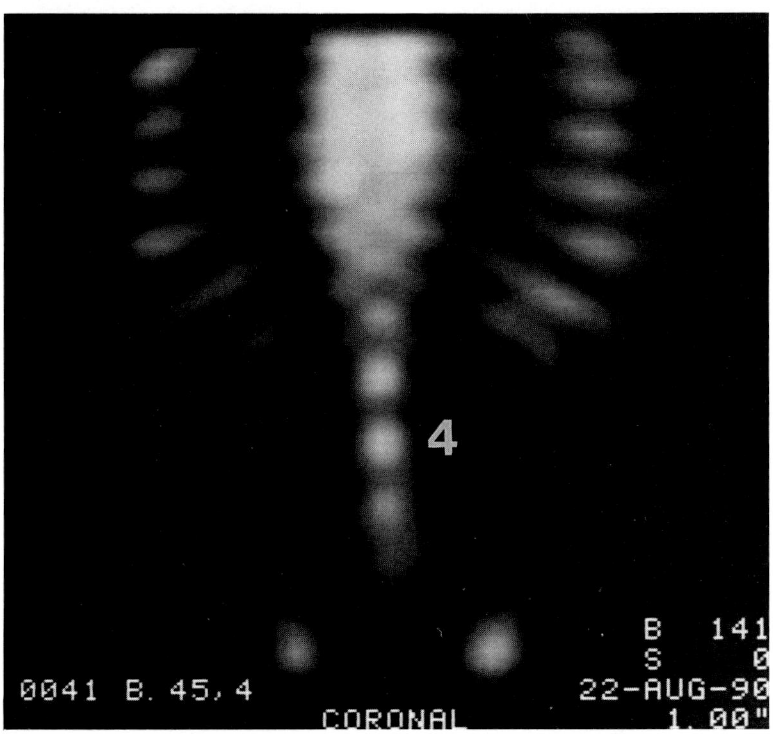

F

(Figure 2.9., cont.)

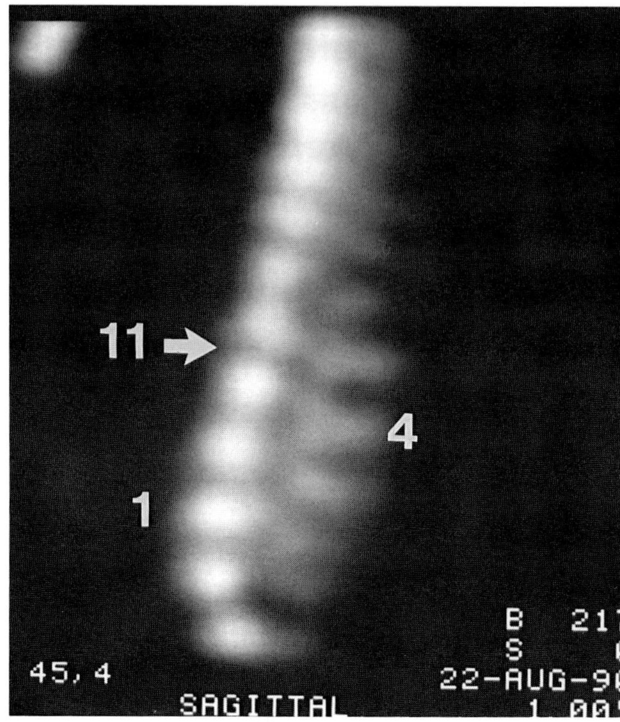

G

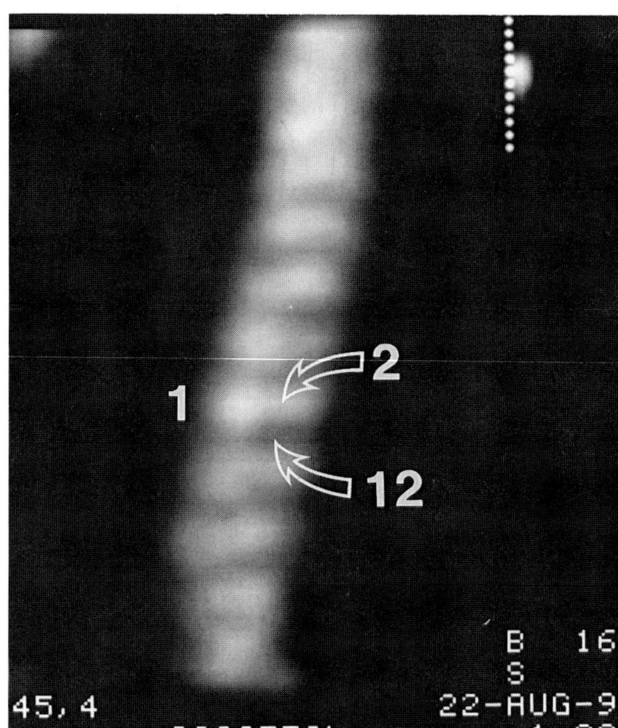

H

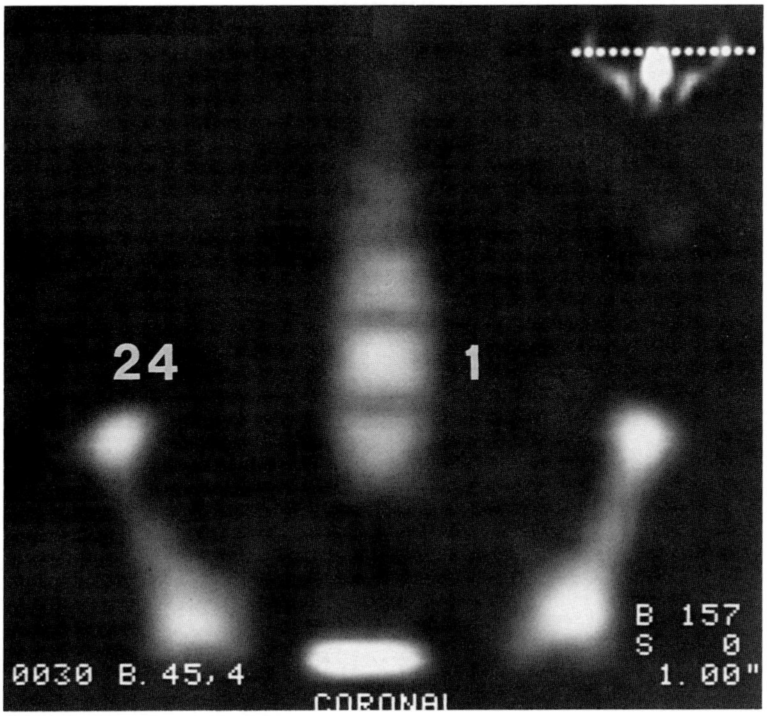

A

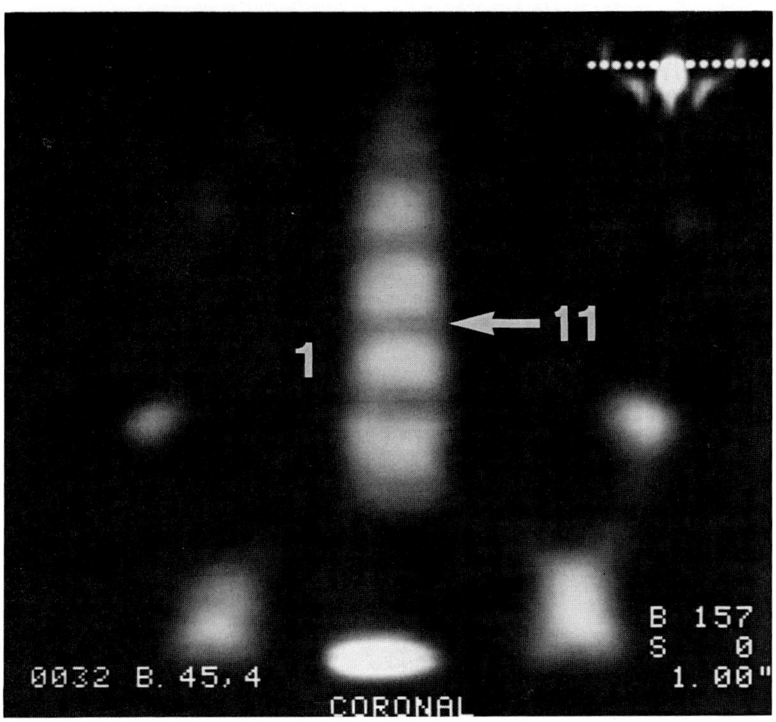

B

Figure 2.10. Lumbar spine (coronal, sagittal, and transverse).

Serial anterior to posterior coronal sections (**A–G**) show the transition of vertebral bodies to elements of the vertebral arch. A midline sagittal section (**H**) shows the lordotic curvature and disc spaces whereas a transverse section (**I**) shows vertebral foramen. **Comment:** The relative size of the vertebral bodies versus disc spaces results in especially good visualization and separation of anatomic structures of the lumbar spine. The lumbar lordotic curve may be fairly minimal in some patients, resulting in adjacent vertebral bodies having a more similar appearance on a single coronal SPECT section compared to the thoracic spine. There are no rib articulations as in the thoracic spine, which simplifies the images and helps in their analysis. The major anatomic landmarks of the lumbar vertebrae that should be identifiable on a SPECT study include vertebral body, pedicles, laminae forming the vertebral arch, areas of the apophyseal joints formed by articulating facets of adjacent superior and inferior articular processes, spinous processes, and vertebral foramen. Transverse processes may be difficult to see.

Sagittal SPECT views resemble lateral radiographic tomograms. Midline sections show the individual vertebral bodies with interval disc spaces behind which is the neural canal in its length. Spinal processes are the most posterior bony structures seen in the midline sagittal views. Sagittal reconstructions to either side of the midline show pedicles and facets.

When viewing coronal reconstructions in an anterior to posterior direction, the lordotic curve of the lumbar spine results in visualization of the lower lumbar vertebral bodies before the upper ones. For this reason, the area of the apophyseal joints of the lower lumbar vertebrae will be viewed in the same coronal plane as the bodies of the upper vertebrae. Sequential anterior to posterior coronal sections show the quad-

Figure 2.10. continued on following page

(Figure 2.10., cont.)

rangular vertebral bodies transforming into the two laterally located, circular-appearing pedicles (Figs. 2.9A–C, 2.10B–D). Further posterior sections show pedicles blending into the superior articular processes and lamina (Figs. 2.9B,C; 2.10D,E); the proximity of these regions plus adjacent inferior articular processes produces an "X" configuration with the base of the spinous processes at the intersection (Figs. 2.9C–E or high on 2.10F). Final posterior SPECT coronal views show laminae merging into spinous processes; the latter is represented by a vertical, linear array of focal sites of tracer activity (Figs. 2.9F; 2.10G).

Transverse sections resemble the familiar computed tomography sections of vertebrae showing body, vertebral foramen, and components of the arch (Fig. 2.9I). The transverse processes may be difficult to see. (Numerical codes are found in the caption of Figure 2.1.)

Figure 2.10. continued on following pages

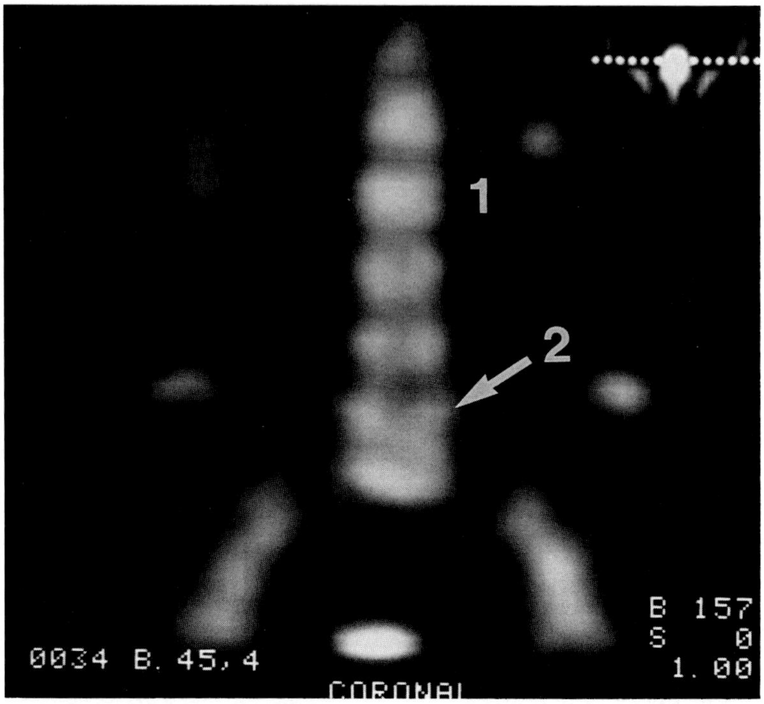

C

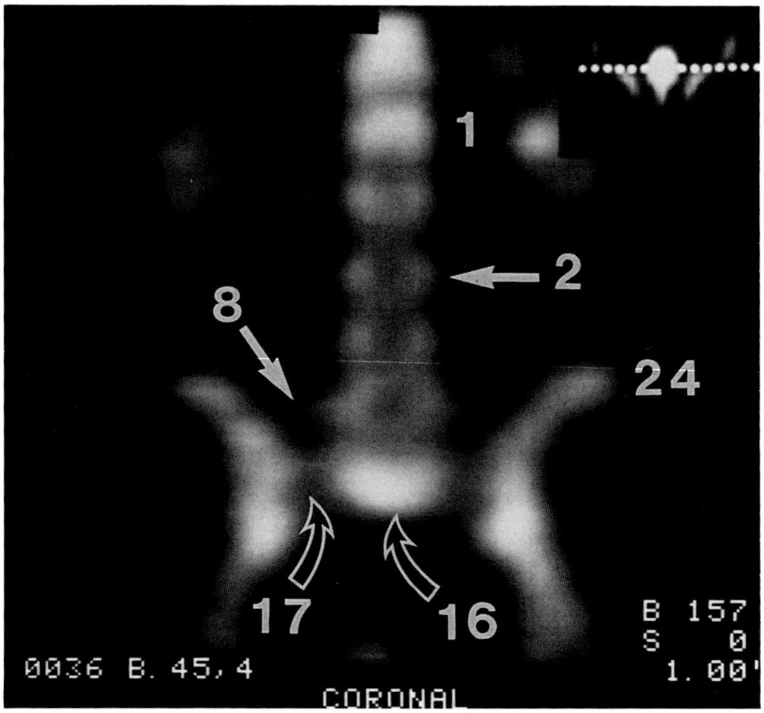

D

(Figure 2.10., cont.)

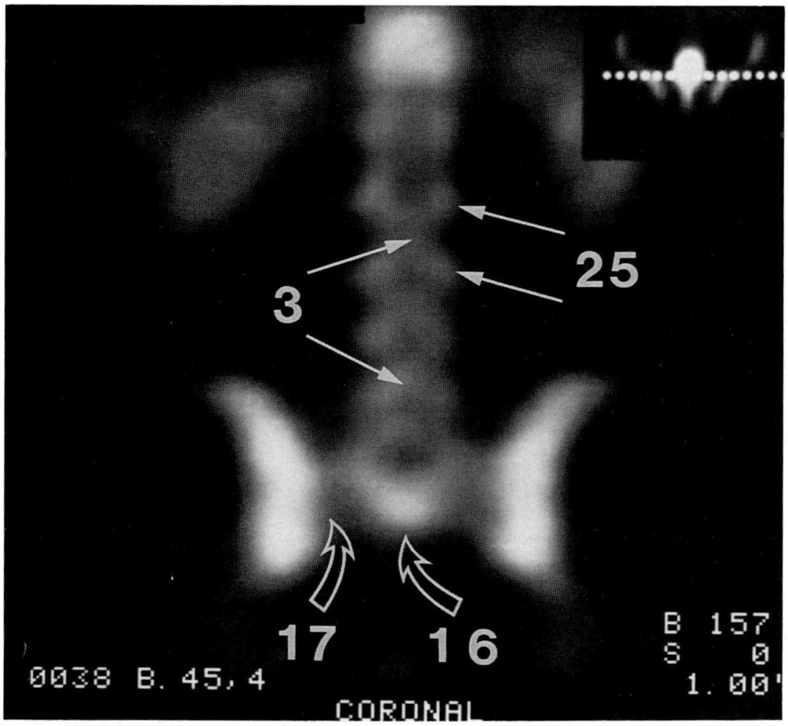

E

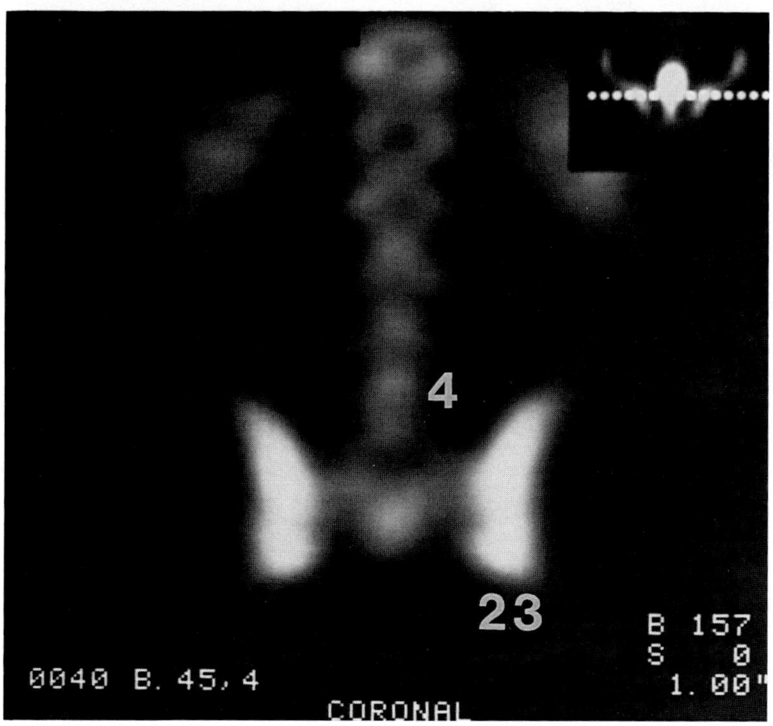

F

(Figure 2.10., cont.)

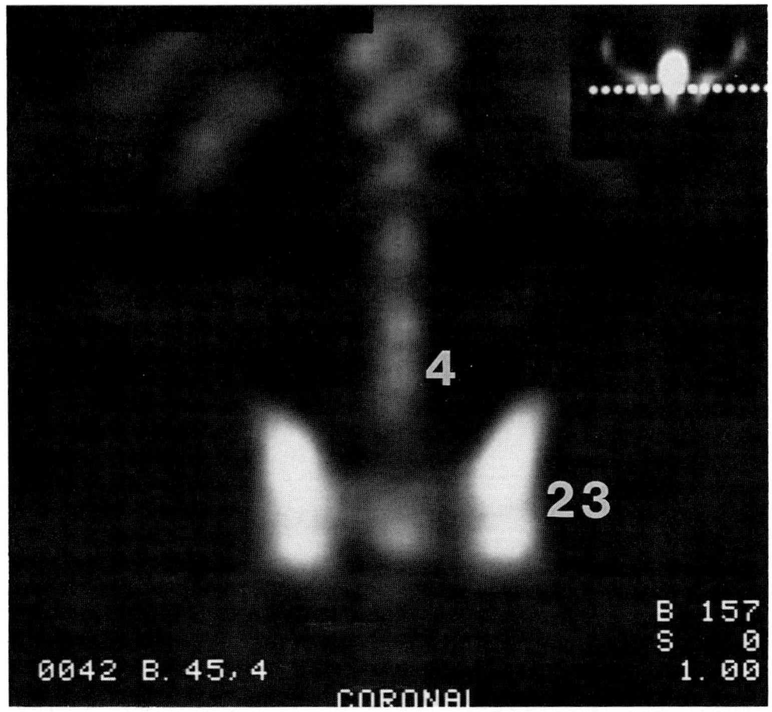

G

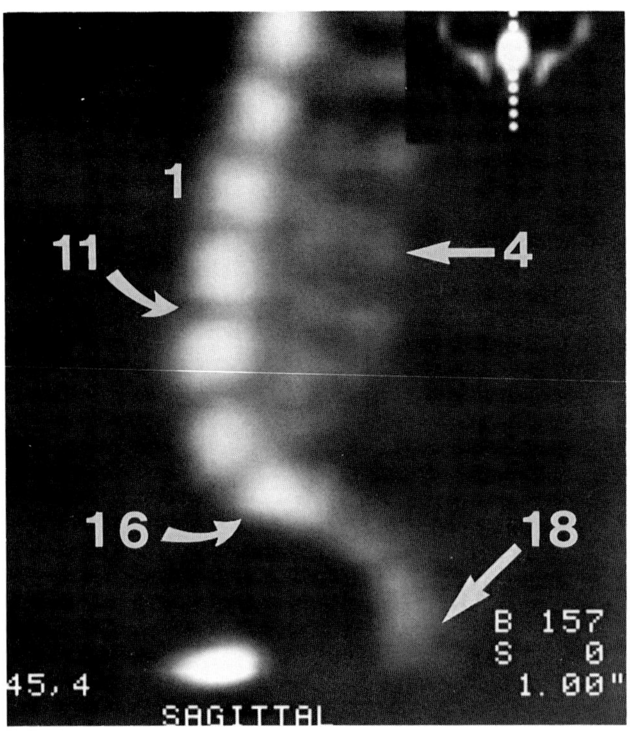

H

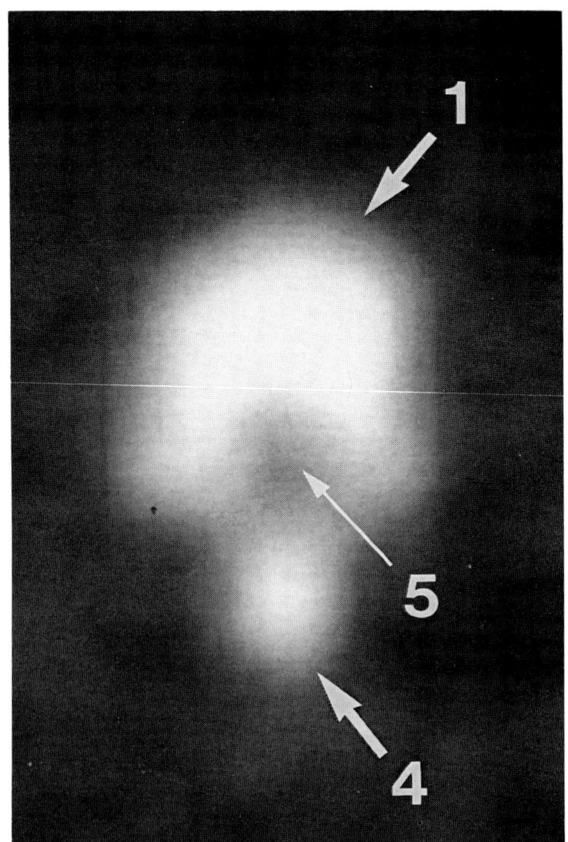

I

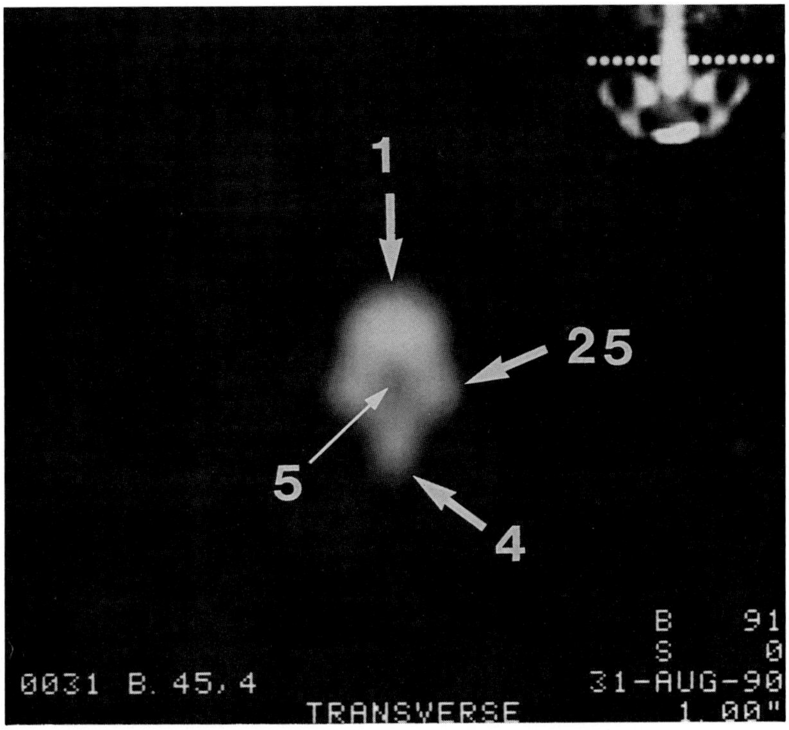

A

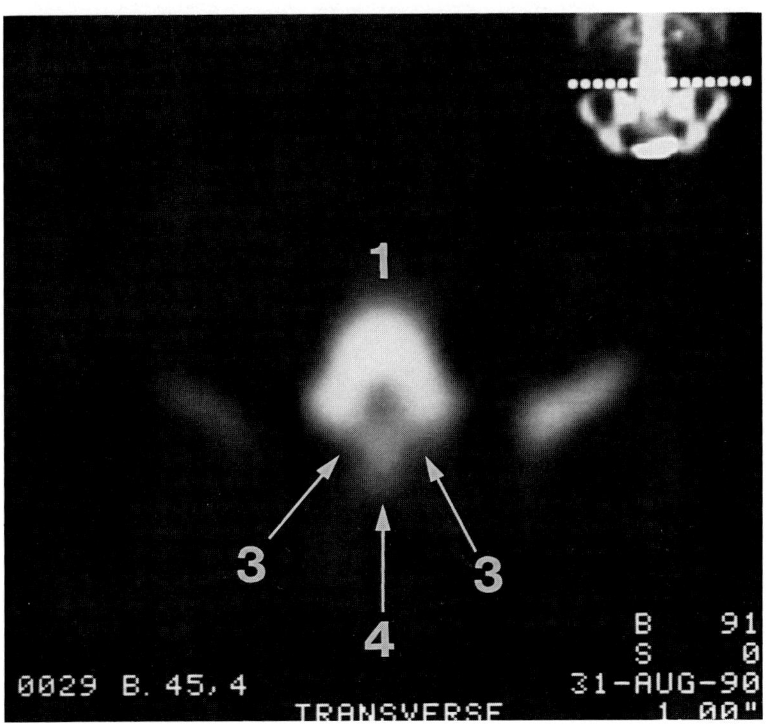

B

Figure 2.11. Sacrococcygeal spine (coronal and transverse).

The normal coronal anatomy of the sacrum with its major components is also illustrated in Fig. 2.10D–G above. In **A** through **H**, sequential transverse sections from the lower lumbar vertebra to sacrum and subsequently coccyx show the normal anatomy of this transition. A sagittal section of the sacrococcygeal spine is shown in Fig. 2.10H.

Comment: A tracer-filled urinary bladder may obscure the sacrococcygeal spine on planar view but separation is possible by SPECT bone scintigraphy. Note that the sacrum with its concave anterior curvature along with the anteriorly directed coccyx are best seen in their entirety on sagittal sections (Fig. 2.10H). Coronal and transverse sections are especially valuable for delineating the sacral ala (Fig. 2.11D) and sacroiliac joints (Figs. 2.11D–G). Occasionally the sacral foramen may be shown on coronal sections, but the vertebral foramen (Fig. 2.11C) is difficult to demonstrate in the lower sacral regions. (Numerical codes are found in the caption of Figure 2.1.)

Figure 2.11. continued on following pages

(Figure 2.11., cont.)

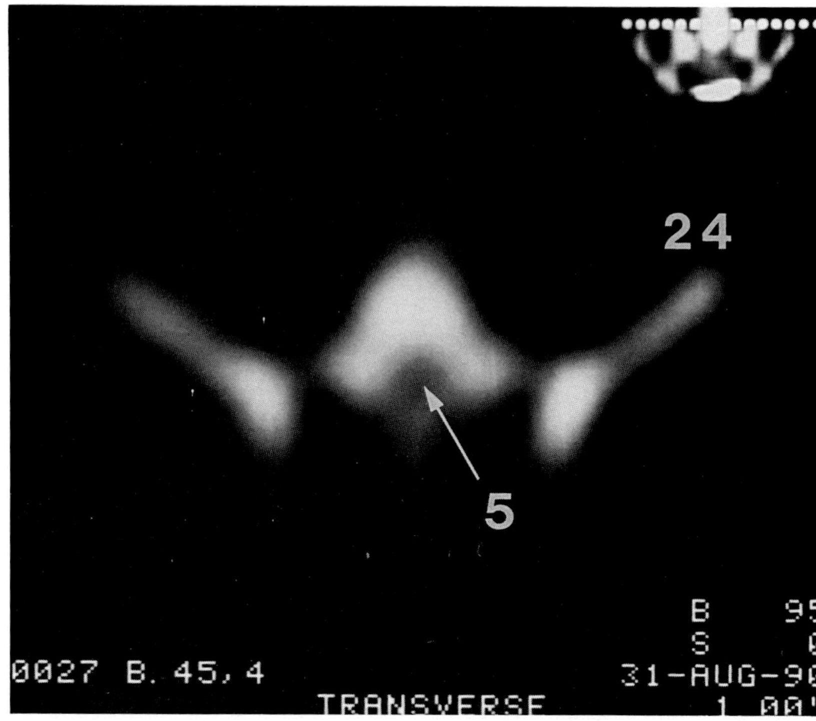

C

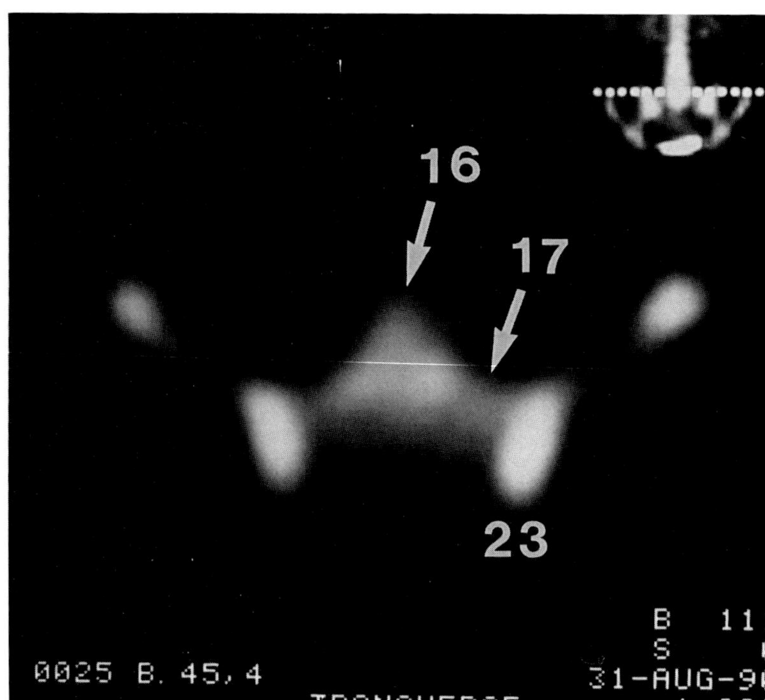

D

(Figure 2.11., cont.)

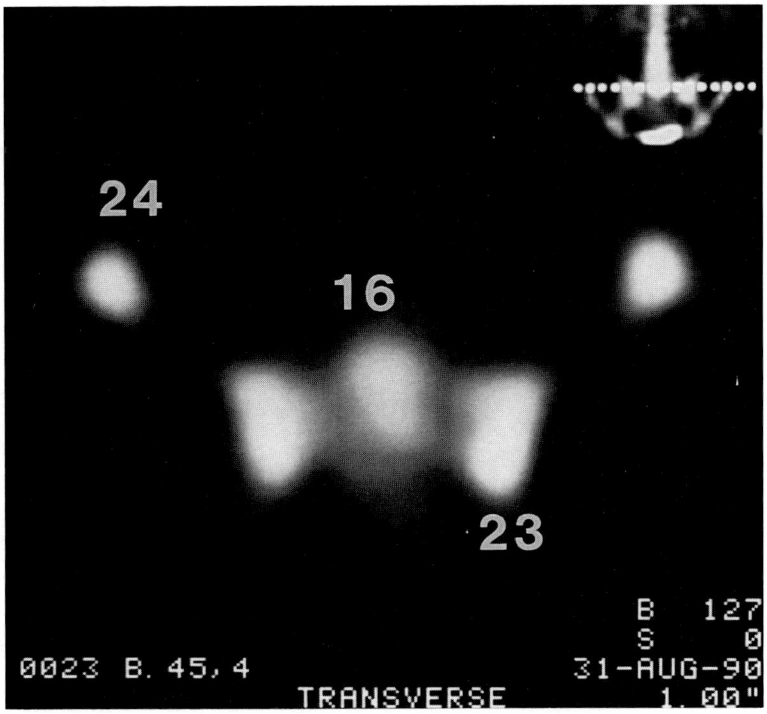

E

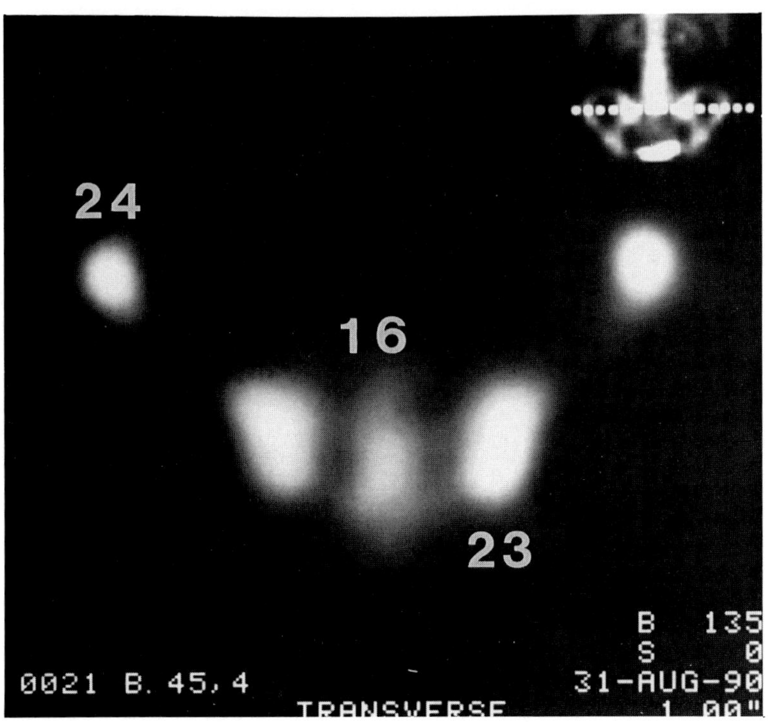

F

(Figure 2.11., cont.)

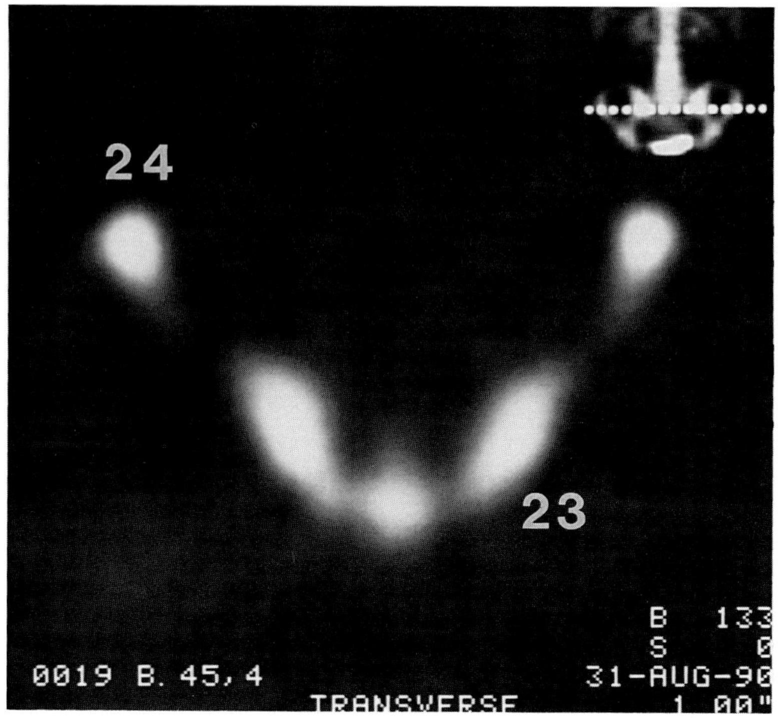

G

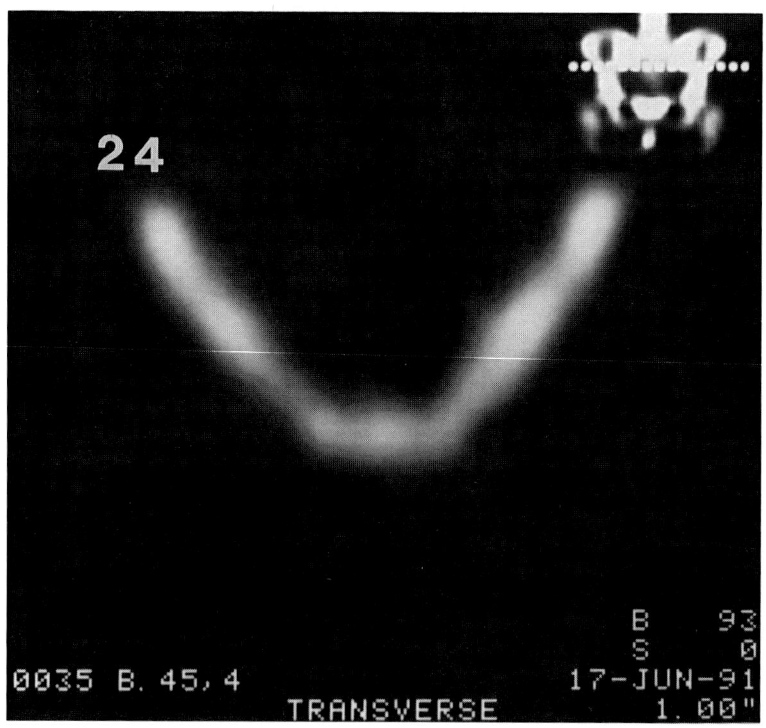

H

The Pelvis and Hips

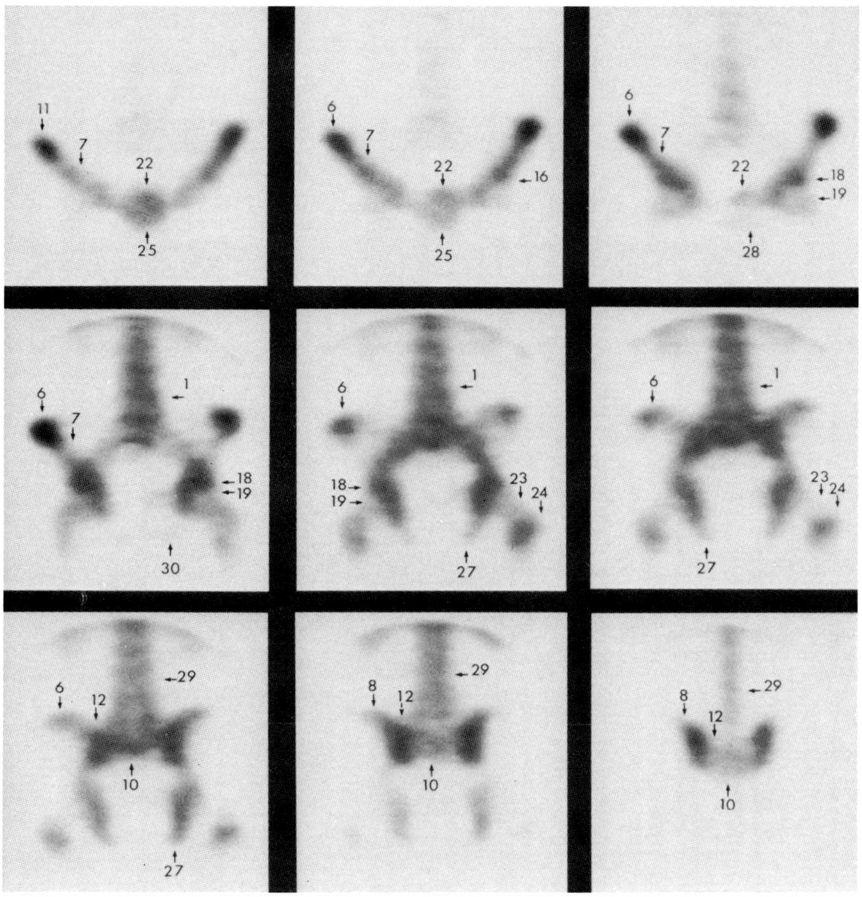

A

Figure 2.12. Pelvis and hips (coronal, sagittal, and transverse).

A: Coronal images from anterior to posterior progressing from left to right and top row to bottom row. **B**: Sagittal images progressing from the left lateral aspect to approximately the midline. **C**: Transverse sections progressing from cranial to caudal. Numerical codes to images:

1. Body of the fifth lumbar vertebrae
2. Spinal canal
3. Pedicle of fifth lumbar vertebrae
4. Lamina of fifth lumbar vertebrae
5. Spinous process of fifth lumbar vertebrae
6. Iliac crest
7. Wing of ilium
8. Ilium
9. Wing of sacrum
10. Sacrum
11. Anterior superior iliac spine
12. Sacroiliac joint
13. Arcuate line
14. Posterior inferior iliac spine
15. Lateral sacral crest
16. Anterior inferior iliac spine
17. Body of ilium
18. Acetabulum
19. Head of the femur
20. Body of ischium
21. Coccyx
22. Urinary bladder
23. Neck of femur
24. Greater trochanter
25. Body of pubis
26. Femoral shaft
27. Ischial tuberosity
28. Inferior ramus of pubis
29. Lumbar spine
30. Ramus of ischium

Figure 2.12. continued on following page

(Figure 2.12., cont.)

Comment: Preparation of the patient for SPECT is important. The patient is instructed to empty the urinary bladder immediately before the study since technical pitfalls due to filling of the bladder affect the quality of the SPECT study. Proper positioning of the patient is also important since shifting or rotation of the pelvis are the cause of asymmetry on SPECT images. This makes interpretation difficult and may lead to false results.

Figure 2.12. continued on following page

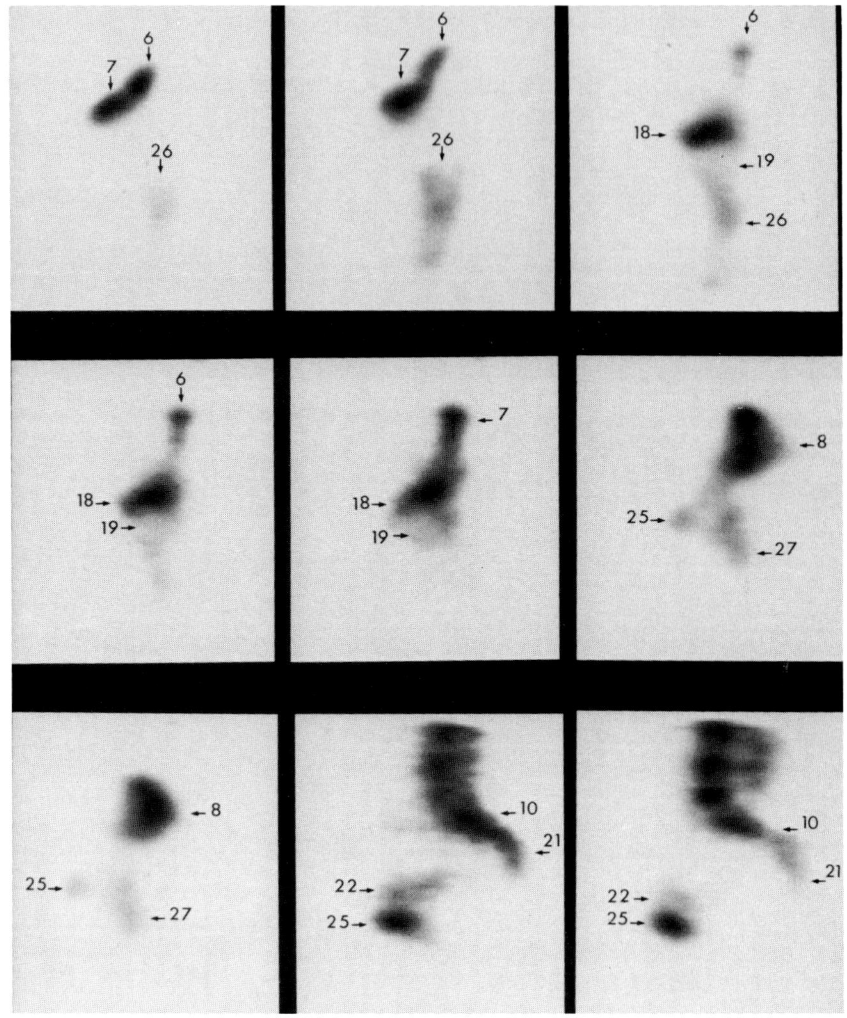

B

(Figure 2.12., cont.)

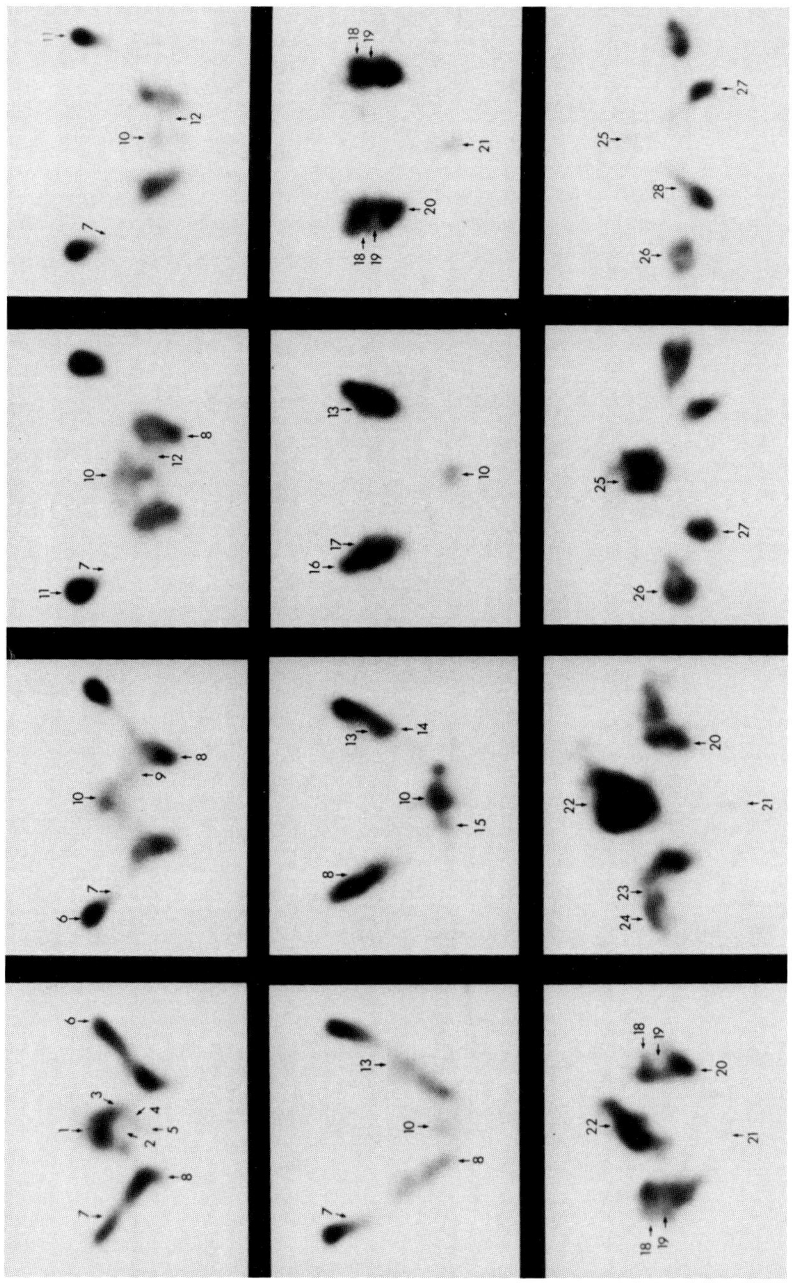

C

Figure 2.13. Avascular necrosis (femoral head – early stage).

Although this is an atlas of the normal SPECT skeletal anatomy, this figure demonstrates abnormal uptake in the femoral head in order that one may better appreciate the normal anatomy. The anterior (*left*) and the posterior (*right*) planar images of the hips (**A**) demonstrate a relative photon deficiency in the femoral head, which was secondary to avascular necrosis (early stage).

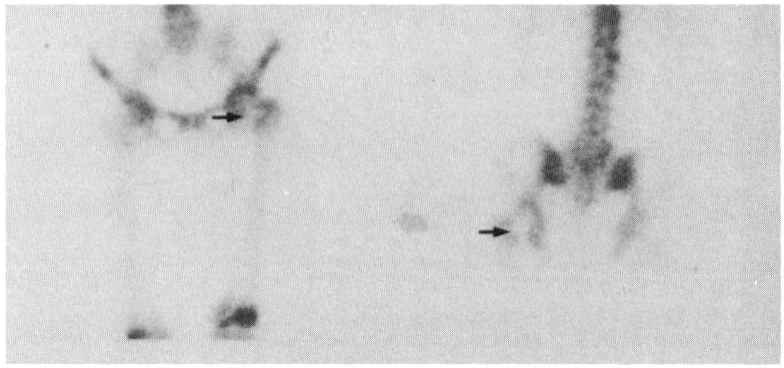

A

Figure 2.13. continued on following page

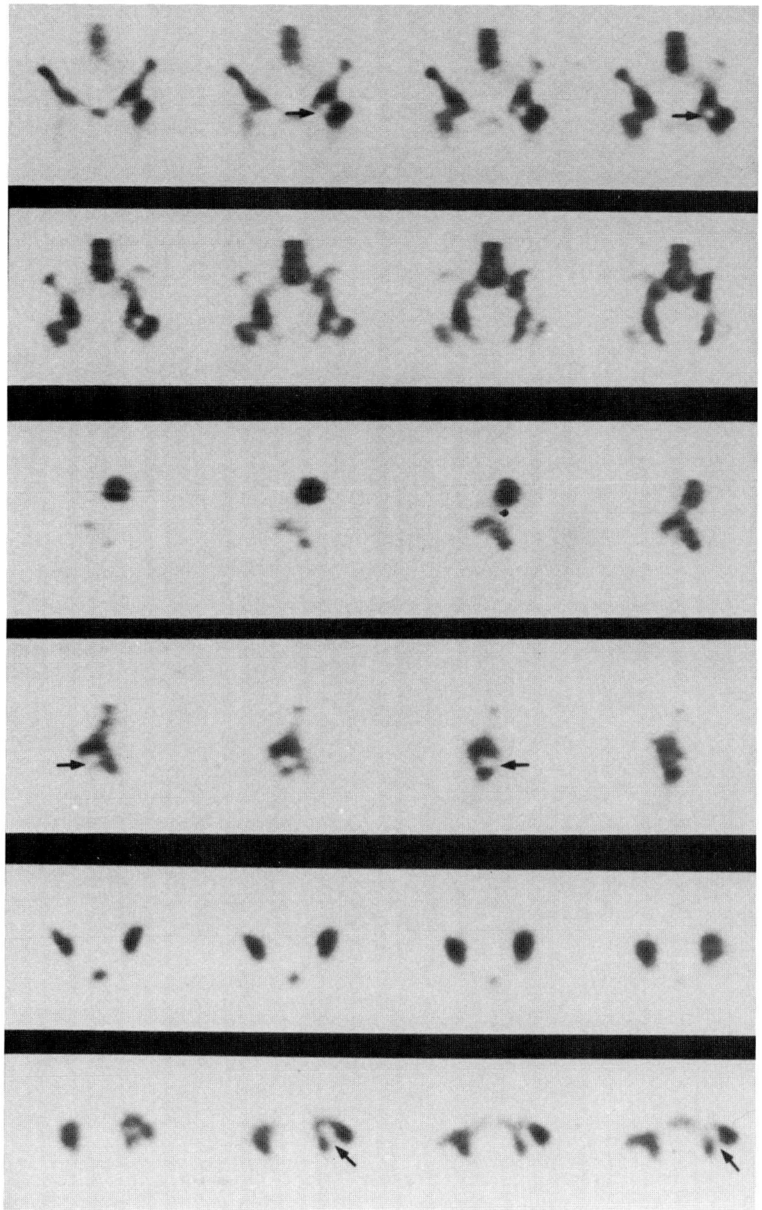

B

(Figure 2.13., cont.)

The SPECT images (**B**) better delineate the photon deficiency in the femoral head (*arrows*). The first two rows are the coronal images, the middle two rows are the sagittal images, and the last two rows are the transverse images. This may be the pattern observed in avascular necrosis shortly after trauma.

Comment: This photon deficiency in the femoral head due to avascular necrosis should be distinguished from the subtle decreased radioactivity in a normal femoral head (Fig. 2.12).

The Skull

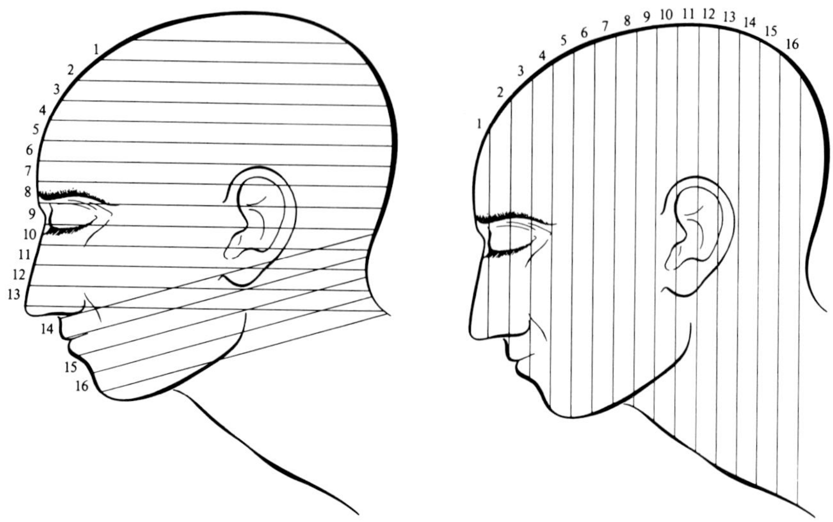

Figure 2.14. Schematic diagram of position of cross-sectional slices.

Left: The various levels of the transverse cross-sectional images, which are number coded and correspond to the levels in the images of Figs. 2.15 and 2.16. **Right:** The various levels of the coronal cross-sectional images, which are also number coded and correspond to the levels in the images of Figs. 2.15 and 2.16. The abbreviations for the anatomical structures in Figs. 2.15 and 2.16 are:

A	atlas
C	cerebellum
E	ethmoid bone
F	frontal bone
FS	frontal sinus
MP	mastoid process
M	mandible
Mar	maxillary alveolar ridge
MS	maxillary sinus
NE	nasal ethmoid bone
O	occipital bone
Opi	internal occipital protuberance
Or	orbit
P	parietal bone
SC	spinal canal
S	sphenoid bone
SS	sphenoid sinus
T	temporal bone
Za	zygomatic arch
Z	zygomatic bone
Zp	zygomatic process

Comment: The anatomy of facial bones is complex and numerous structures overlap, making accurate location of abnormalities by planar bone scanning extremely difficult. SPECT, which separates structures in three dimensions as already demonstrated, can be especially valuable in the assessment of the facial bones and calvarium. The following images demonstrate the normal anatomy on SPECT bone imaging of the facial bones and calvarium.

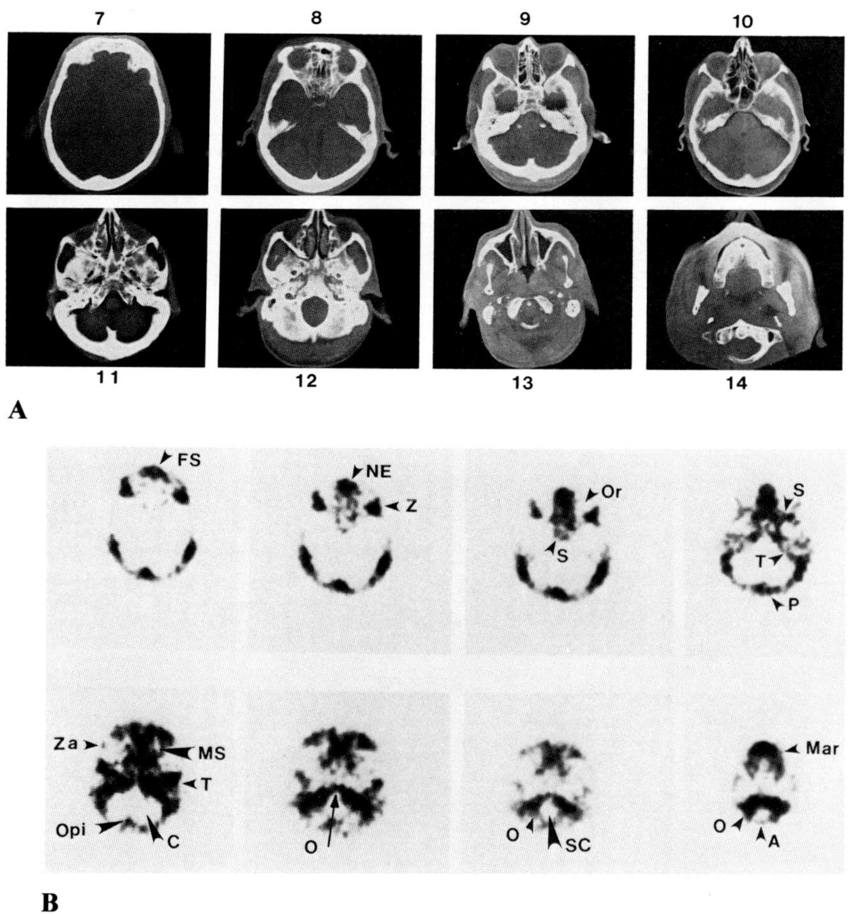

Figure 2.15. Transverse sections.

A: A normal transverse computed axial tomography. The numbered level of each image corresponds to the transverse cross-sections demonstrated in Fig. 2.14 and to the SPECT images in **B**. There is a slight variation due to different slice thickness, head positioning, and angle of cuts. The abbreviations are listed in Fig. 2.14.
(Reprinted with permission from Gambarelli J, Guerinel G, Chevrot L, Mattei M. In: *Computerized Axial Tomography*. New York: Springer-Verlag, NY, 1977, pp. 45–61).

Figure 2.16. Coronal sections.

A: A normal coronal computed axial tomography. The numbered level of each image corresponds to the coronal cross-sections demonstrated in Fig. 2.14 (*right image*) and to the SPECT images in **B**. Abbreviations are listed in Fig. 2.14.
(Reprinted with permission from Gambarelli J, Guerinel G, Chevrot L, Mattei M. In: *Computerized Axial Tomography*. New York: Springer-Verlag, NY, 1977, pp. 69–87).

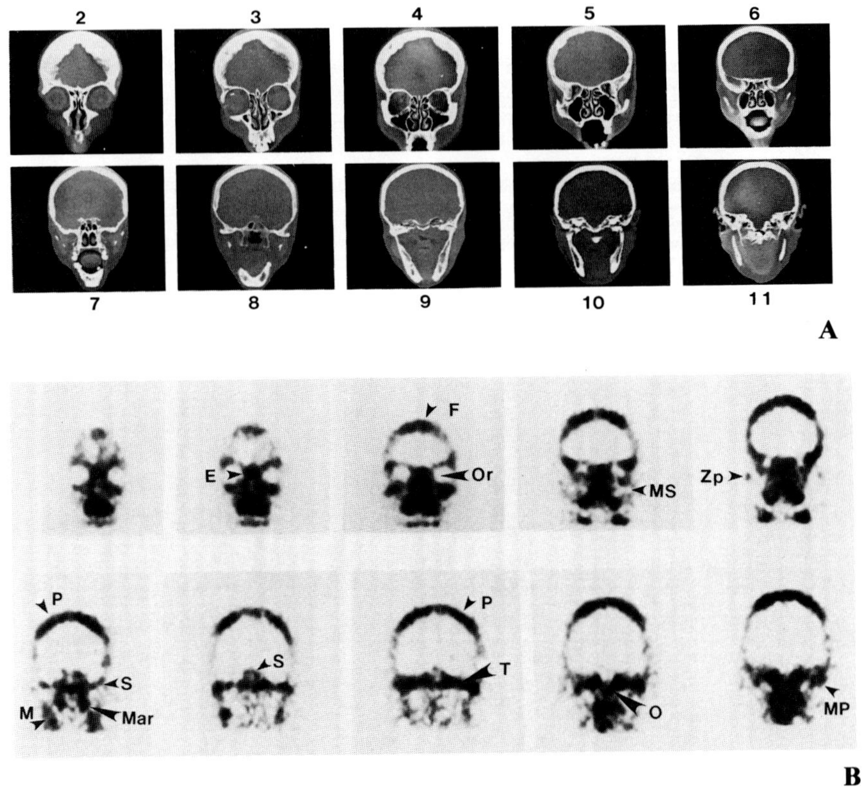

Figure 2.17. Sagittal sections.

Sequential 6-mm sagittal SPECT slices progress from the midline (*upper left*) to the lateral skull (*lower right*). Abbreviations are listed in index for skull illustrations.

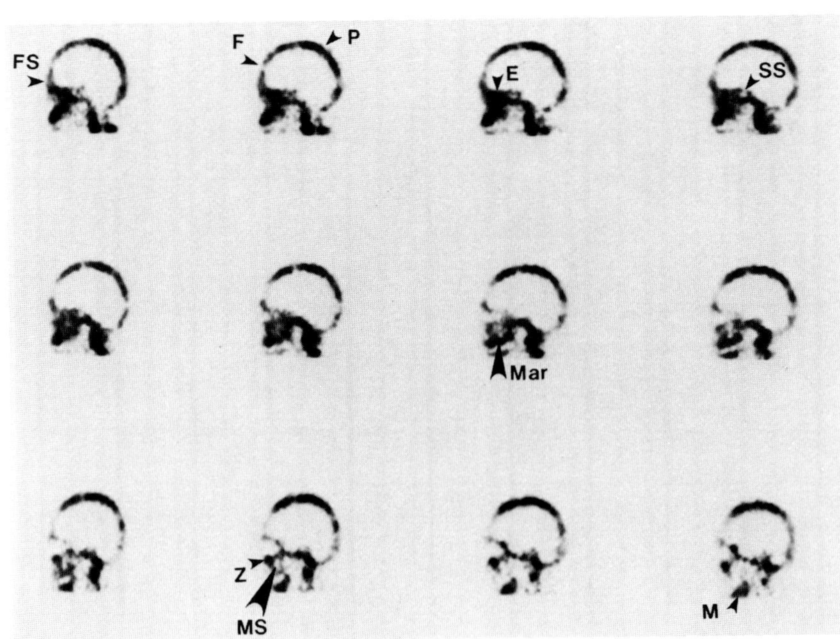

References

1. Gates GF. Normal anatomy of the lumbosacral spine and pelvis: a correlation of SPECT and radiographic techniques. *Clin Nucl Med.* 1988;13:327–330.
2. Gates GF. SPECT imaging of the lumbosacral and pelvis. *Clin Nucl Med.* 1988;13:907–914.
3. Collier BD, Carrera GF, Johnson RP, et al. Detection of femoral head avascular necrosis in adults by SPECT. *J Nucl Med.* 1985;26:979–987.
4. Collier BD, Hellman RS, Krasnow AZ, et al. Bone SPECT. *Semin Nucl Med.* 1987;17:247–266.
5. Weber DA. Options in camera and camera technology for bone scan: role of SPECT. *Semin Nucl Med.* 1988;18:78–89.
6. Israel O, Jerushalmi J, Frenkel A, et al. Normal and abnormal single photon emission computed tomography of the skull: comparison with planar scintigraphy. *J Nucl Med.* 1988;29:1341–1346.
7. Gates GF, Goris ML. Maxillary-facial abnormalities assessed by bone imaging. *Radiology.* 1976;121:677–682.
8. Brown ML, Keyes JW Jr, Leonard PF, et al. Facial bone scanning by emission tomography. *J Nucl Med.* 1977;18:1184–1188.
9. Wallis JW, Miller TR. Volume rendering in three-dimensional display of SPECT images. *J Nucl Med.* 1990;31:1421–1430.

CHAPTER 3

Atlas of SPECT Quality Control and Examples of Artifacts

L. Stephen Graham, Ralph R. Lake, and Marvin B. Cohen

Numerous articles have documented the advantages of Single Photon Emission Computed Tomography (SPECT) in a wide variety of clinical studies.[1-4] The production of high quality diagnostic studies demands the highest performance from the camera and computer and careful attention to detail by the technologist conducting the study. Scintillation cameras with minor nonuniformities may give satisfactory planar images but if used for SPECT imaging may produce images that provide less diagnostic information or even create false positives.[5,6] The purpose of this chapter is to describe a quality control (QC) program, to recommend the appropriate frequencies for performing quality control tests, and to provide examples of common problems. The following topics will be discussed: X and Y axes calibration, center-of-rotation, field uniformity correction, and phantoms.

X and Y Axes Calibration

If the pixels in a SPECT image are not the same size in both dimensions, then accurate coronal and sagittal reconstructions will not be obtained. Unequal dimensions will also produce distorted images when the X and Y axes are rotated to generate images that are perpendicular to the major axis of the heart.[6] In addition, a change in pixel size may produce inaccuracies in attenuation correction.

Many SPECT systems have software that guides the user through the process of calibrating pixel size. If such software is not available, two point sources can be sequentially positioned along the X and Y axes at a known distance of separation and the number of pixels per mm or cm calculated. A difference of more than 5%, or whatever is specified by the vendor, in the two dimensions requires an adjustment that is usually done by service personnel. Because of its importance, it is generally recommended that this calibration be performed on a monthly basis.[7,8]

Center-of-Rotation

The purpose of a center-of-rotation calibration is to provide congruence between the center of the camera image and the center of the computer matrix. In most systems a set of correction factors are calculated from the data acquired during this procedure. Before reconstruction, offset corrections are applied to individual views to produce congruence.

A consistent offset error as small as 3.2 mm for a 64 × 64 matrix (no zoom) can produce a 30% loss of spatial resolution and a 40% loss of contrast.[9] Larger errors produce markedly greater losses of spatial resolution (Fig. 3.1) and contrast and can produce a clinical image that bears little resemblance to the organ being studied (Fig. 3.2).

A center-of-rotation calibration must be carried out on a regular basis. The general consensus is that this procedure should be carried out once each week.[6–8,10] If more frequent calibrations are required to maintain satisfactory operation of a SPECT system, service personnel should be called to determine the cause of the instability.

The procedure for acquiring a center-of-rotation calibration varies markedly from vendor to vendor. Some require the use of a point source, and other vendors require a line. Some require that the source be located on or near the axis of rotation, the imaginary line around which the camera rotates. Others specify that the source be positioned off-axis. Regardless of the specific methodology, all systems require that a separate center-of-rotation be performed for each collimator that is used for SPECT studies. Most also require a separate center-of-rotation when zoom mode (magnification) is used. Some even require that a center-of-rotation be acquired for different matrix sizes.

From the standpoint of spatial resolution, high quality SPECT studies are obtained when the center-of-rotation does not change significantly with projection angle in systems that use an average value for the center-of-rotation. Information about the center-of-rotation as a function of angle is readily available in most systems by reviewing the output of the center-of-rotation analysis program (Fig 3.3). These diagrams and other quantitative information that are provided must be carefully examined to identify potential problems.

Parellelism of Collimator Holes

Having performed a center-of-rotation calibration, it can generally be assumed that congruence between the camera image and computer matrix is assured. There are two reasons why that may not be the case. First, the center-of-rotation calibration assumes that all holes in the collimator are parallel to one another. During data collection only a small portion of the collimator actually "sees" a point source. As a result, the correction factor that is calculated is an average over the portion of the collimator that is used. Any variation in hole angulation of the "unused" portions of the collimator produces regional losses of spatial resolution. The general consensus is that hole angle variation should not exceed 0.25° to 0.5°.[11]

A rigorous test of hole angulation requires a special setup and special software.[11–13] However, a qualitative evaluation is easy to perform.[14,15] With the collimator to be tested pointing horizontally, a source of approximately 5 mCi should be positioned at a distance of 3.5 to 5 meters. The radioactive source or camera head must then be adjusted until the image is centered in the field of view. Two and a half million counts are sufficient to provide an image for checking collimator hole angulation (see Fig. 3.4). A satisfactory collimator will produce an image that is radially symmetric, that is, the intensity will decrease uniformly in all directions as you move out from the central region of high intensity (Fig.

3.4A). Small striations are acceptable (Fig. 3.4B) but large variations such as those shown in Figure 3.4C are not.

Alignment of Conjugate Views

The second problem, which may occur despite good center-of-rotation calibrations, is relatively uncommon but should be evaluated periodically. If the detector assembly is not aligned so that it moves radially relative to the axis of rotation, the center-of-rotation calibration will be correct only for the radius of rotation used for the calibration. A simple test can be used to verify detector alignment. Perform a SPECT study on a straight line of radioactivity with a different radius than the one used for center-of-rotation calibration, preferably with a 128 $\times$ 128 matrix. Then reconstruct the data with a ramp filter. A transverse slice should appear as a gaussian-shaped point. Any image that appears otherwise should be discussed with service personnel. Detector misalignment will show the same types of errors as those presented in Figure 3.1.

Field Uniformity Correction

Many SPECT clinical studies require renormalization by high count (30–120M) floods. The basis for this requirement is quite simple. In state-of-the-art scintillation cameras, the intrinsic (collimator removed) integral uniformity as measured using the National Electrical Manufacturers Association (NEMA) protocol with ^{99m}Tc is no better than 2% and in some cameras may exceed 4%. When the collimator and scatter are added, the uniformity is considerably poorer, often on the order of 5% to 6%. Yet it has been documented that when high count images are acquired, small nonuniformities >1% produce "ring" (Figs. 3.5 and 3.6) or "crescent" artifacts.[16] Large nonuniformities and those that are not near the axis of rotation will produce less dramatic rings.[17]

High count density SPECT studies may show ring artifacts (Fig. 3.7). However, clinical SPECT studies that contain low count density such as those involving the administration of ^{201}Tl to evaluate myocardial perfusion may not exhibit these artifacts because they are washed out by statistical fluctuations in radioactive decay and the reconstruction process.

Most references recommend that floods for renormalization be acquired once each week and that daily QC films be carefully scrutinized. Each vendor's protocol for acquisition of these floods must be carefully followed. As with center-of-rotation calibration, high count floods are needed for each collimator used for SPECT and for zoom mode. Use of high count flood renormalization ("flood field correction") does not guarantee the production of SPECT images without ring or crescent artifacts. Renormalization may not correct for marked nonuniformity because it does not correct for nonlinearity, the primary cause of nonuniformity (Fig. 3.8).

State-of-the-art cameras are extremely variable with respect to the effect of changes in photon energy on the production of nonuniformity. In general, cameras that do not use light pipes, contoured pieces of lucite positioned between the glass plates that cover the crystal and the photomultiplier tubes, are more likely to produce a nonuniform image when radionuclides such as ^{201}Tl, ^{111}In, and ^{67}Ga are used (Fig. 3.9). The visibility of these artifacts is determined by the amplitude of the nonuniformity and the count density of the image.

Angular Sampling

It may appear logical to conclude that performing the calibrations that have just been described guarantees a high quality, artifact-free image. Unfortunately, that is not the case. Choices that are made relative to data acquisition and those made before reconstruction have a dramatic effect on the appearance of the final image. To avoid the production of significant streak artifacts, at least 60 views (angular samples) must be acquired. The same angular sampling in 180° ^{201}Tl studies is achieved with 30 views. Even with 60 views in a 360° study, local areas of high activity may increase the intensity of streaks to the point where other structures are obscured. This is often the case when pelvic structures are obscured by activity in the bladder,[18] when the spleen has high uptake (Fig. 3.10), and when a region of high activity is produced by extravasation of tracer during injection. These artifacts can be reduced by using 120 or even 180 views.

Matrix Size

In addition to using satisfactory angular sampling, linear sampling (matrix size) must be adequate. For studies of organs that are stationary, either 64 × 64 or 128 × 128 matrices can be used. The choice depends on the organ to be imaged. Although some users recommend the use of 128 × 128 matrices for bone studies, which is consistent with the sampling theorem, some references indicate 64 × 64 is adequate.[18]

The choice of matrix size is not simple when high resolution images are needed. For structures that are not moving, the collimator that is used is an important variable. The size of a pixel must be between one-half and one-third the full width at half maximum (FWHM) of the system (detector plus collimator) spatial resolution. The FWHM is determined by the collimator that is being used and the radius of rotation. When the pixel size meets the condition described above and the radius of rotation is as small as possible, image contrast will be improved.

Phantoms

It is often recommended that a phantom be used for SPECT quality control on a periodic basis.[5-8,18] Recommended frequencies range from monthly to semiannually. The value of these studies lies in the ability to test SPECT systems under conditions that simulate clinical conditions. Because the nature of the object is fully known, the reconstructed images can be reviewed for the presence of unsuspected ring or crescent artifacts, spatial resolution losses, inaccuracies in attenuation correction, and loss of contrast. Although the subject is not covered in this chapter, studies with a phantom can also be used to evaluate the effect of different acquisition and processing parameters.[19]

Commercial Phantoms

The most commonly used phantoms are presented in Figure 3.11. Both contain a uniform section, one with cold or hot spheres for evaluating contrast, and some type of resolution pattern.

Protocol for Performance Testing of SPECT Systems

Even though numerous authors recommend periodic studies with a phantom, few provide information on the setup and processing parameters to be used. Furthermore, methods for evaluating the results are seldom discussed. The protocol presented in Table 3.1 can be used to provide images that are useful in evaluating overall SPECT system performance.

Evaluation of Attenuation Correction

A transverse reconstruction of a uniform section can be used to evaluate a number of parameters. First, the accuracy of attenuation correction should be assessed. A five pixel wide profile drawn in the X and Y direction should be flat except for variations due to statistical fluctuations and reconstruction noise (Fig. 3.12). Reduced intensity in the center relative to the edge indicates undercorrection; a high intensity in the center indicates overcorrection. A profile that is essentially a straight line but is tilted (positive or negative slope) indicates an attenuation boundary that was improperly drawn (Fig. 3.12). Profiles that show under or over correction for attenuation may be caused by a) incorrect pixel size calibration, b) use of the wrong attenuation coefficient, c) software errors, d) change in energy resolution of the camera, e) incorporation of hardware or software techniques for removing scattered photons. Improper attenuation correction can have a significant impact on the appearance of clinical studies (Fig. 3.12E).

Qualitative Evaluation of Uniformity

The same transverse section can also be used to assess uniformity and/or noise qualitatively or quantitatively. Qualitatively, the image should not show ring or crescent artifacts even without the application of a high count flood correction. If artifacts are present, they should disappear when flood correction is applied (see Fig. 3.13). The general appearance

Table 3.1. Protocol for performance testing of a SPECT system.

1. Mount the general purpose collimator on the detector
2. Fill a Data Spectrum Corporation or Nuclear Associates phantom with a uniform solution of ^{99m}Tc containing approximately eight mCi (12 mCi if a high resolution collimator is used)
3. Fasten the phantom to the end of the imaging table, taking care that the phantom is aligned parallel to the axis of rotation in both directions
4. Set a symmetric 20% window on the photopeak of ^{99m}Tc
5. Set the detector so that the average radius of rotation is 20 cm
6. Acquire a 60 (64)-view 360° SPECT study using a 64 × 64 matrix and 200K counts/view (if a rectangular or jumbo field-of-view camera is used the image must be magnified so the pixel size is between 6.0 and 7.0 mm)
7. Reconstruct the data set with a Hann filter at 1 Nyquist or its equivalent (see Table 3.2)

of the image should be similar to that of a benchmark study that was performed after acceptance tests were completed.

Quantitative Evaluation of Uniformity

If desired, quantitative measurements of uniformity can be made. All SPECT systems provide standard keyboard commands that can be used to make these measurements. Some provide data that can be used to calculate noise as well. A 15 × 15 pixel square (225 pixels) region-of-interest (ROI) must be drawn in the center of the image of the phantom (Fig. 3.14). In many systems, the ROI statistics will include the maximum and minimum, average, and in some cases the standard deviation. If the minimum is not included, the lower threshold can be raised to reveal more clearly the "coolest" pixel. A one-pixel ROI can then be used to obtain the number of counts in that pixel. These data can be used to calculate two performance parameters from the following equations:

$$\text{Uniformity} = \frac{(\text{Maximum pixel count} - \text{Minimum pixel count})}{(\text{Maximum pixel count} + \text{Minimum pixel count})} \times 100$$

$$\text{Root mean square (RMS) noise} = \frac{\text{Standard deviation for ROI}}{\text{Average pixel count}} \times 100$$

Of course the latter can be calculated only if the standard deviation is given for the square ROI by the computer software. These values can be compared to those presented in Table 3.3 provided the protocol for data acquisition and processing given in Tables 3.1 and 3.2 is carefully followed.

Qualitative and Quantitative Evaluation of Contrast

Contrast can be evaluated from the transverse section that most clearly shows the spheres. If only qualitative information is desired, simply note the number of spheres that can be visualized and compare the image to a benchmark film (Fig. 3.15). Quantitative data can be obtained by finding the number of counts in the "coolest" pixel in the regions associated with

Table 3.2. Reconstruction filters and cutoff values for SPECT phantom performance study.

Computer	Filter name	Cutoff
ADAC	Hamming	1 Nyquist
Elscint	Hann	Parameter a = 0 Parameter b = 1 Parameter c = 1
General Electric	Hann	0.76/cm[a]
Picker PCS512	Filter 3	
Siemens MaxiDelta	Shepp & Logan/Hann	1 Nyquist
Sophy	Hann	1 Nyquist
Toshiba	Chesler	1 Nyquist
Spectrum	Hamming/Hann	1 Nyquist

[a]Cutoff calculated for pixel size of 0.64 cm. For other pixel sizes, the cutoff must be calculated as described in the vendor's procedure manual.

each sphere. In some systems an ROI drawn over each sphere (Fig. 3.16) will provide statistics that include the minimum pixel counts. If such information is not provided it can be found by eliminating the display of low count values (thresholding) to clarify the location of the coolest pixel within a sphere. Then, a one-pixel ROI can be used to obtain the actual number of counts. Contrast can be calculated using the equation:

$$\text{Contrast} = \frac{(\text{Average pixel counts} - \text{Minimum pixel counts})}{\text{Average pixel counts}} \times 100$$

The average pixel counts is the average number of counts per pixel obtained from the 15 × 15 pixel ROI set on the uniform transverse section. Acceptable values are shown in Table 3.3.

It must be emphasized that several variables can produce contrast values that fall outside the values presented in Table 3.3. A wide window (>20%) will include more scatter and decrease contrast. Conversely, a window narrower than 20% will increase contrast. Any technique that removes scatter, such as energy-weighted-acquisition, will also increase contrast. Use of a low resolution collimator will produce low contrast values.

Qualitative Evaluation of Resolution

An estimate of spatial resolution can be obtained by adding together 10 transverse slices that cut through the cold rods in the lower part of the phantom (Fig. 3.17). The resulting image can be compared to a benchmark film. Although this technique can be useful for monitoring spatial resolution, it is critically dependent on using the same acquisition and processing parameters each time and the phantom must be perfectly parallel to the axis of rotation.

Summary

SPECT studies have clearly demonstrated the ability to provide information that is not available from planar images. But this will be true only when all aspects of the camera from basic camera performance to data acquisition and the selection of reconstruction parameters are carefully selected and controlled. Of necessity, this requires a comprehensive quality control program.

The importance of regular center-of-rotation calibration cannot be

Table 3.3. Acceptable uniformity, noise, and contrast values for SPECT system performance study.

Parameters	Acceptable values (%)
Sphere contrast	
31.8 mm	56–83
25.4 mm	35–56
19.1 mm	20–42
15.4 mm	5–36
Uniformity	19–28
RMS noise	7–11

overemphasized. Ring or crescent artifacts produced by nonuniformities may produce false positives, although the pattern can be recognized by the astute and knowledgeable physician. The loss of spatial resolution associated with center-of-rotation errors is much more subtle and unless it is quite large, produces a pattern that can easily be overlooked.

All users must be familiar with the artifacts that may appear in SPECT studies.[5] Regardless of how frequently QC procedures are done, there is no guarantee that malfunctions or failures will not occur just before the time clinical studies are performed.

Atlas Section

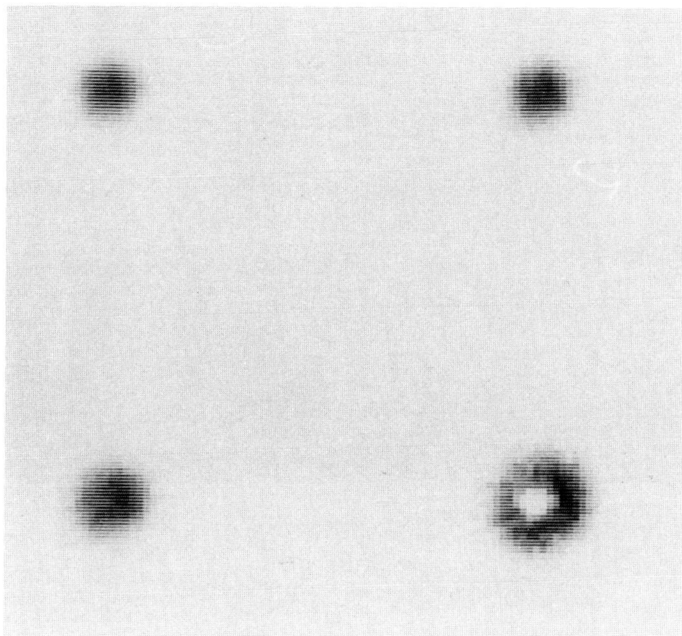

Figure 3.1. Center of rotation: quality control.

Four SPECT transverse section images (128 × 128) of a line source reconstructed with a Ramp filter are demonstrated with various errors of center of rotation. The image in the upper left has no significant center of rotation error. The image in the upper right has an average uncorrected center-of-rotation error of 0.4 pixel. Note a slight increase in size of the image. The FWHM increased by 15% relative to the image with no center-of-rotation error. The image in the lower left has an average uncorrected center-of-rotation error of 0.9 pixel. Image size is increased significantly. The FWHM is larger by 30% than the image with no error. The image in the lower right has an average uncorrected center-of-rotation error of 2.4 pixels. Note the lack of symmetry and appearance of a central cold region.

Comment: 1. If the detector assembly is not aligned so that it moves radially 180°, the center-of-rotation calibration will be correct only for the radius of rotation used in the center-of-rotation calibration. Errors in detector alignment will also appear as above. 2. Assuring good center-of-rotation calibration is very important to SPECT imaging, but the physician cannot rely on determining if adequate center-of-rotation calibration is present by reviewing the patient images. Although the physician may easily identify large calibration errors, such images may have little resemblance to the organ studied (as in Fig. 3.2), and the physician will not be able to identify small calibrations errors, which may result either in poor quality images with reduced resolution, contrast, and diagnostic yield or in artifacts, which the physician may intepret as disease. Center-of-rotation calibration must be done on a routine basis, which is discussed earlier in the chapter.

Figure 3.2. Center of rotation: clinical example.

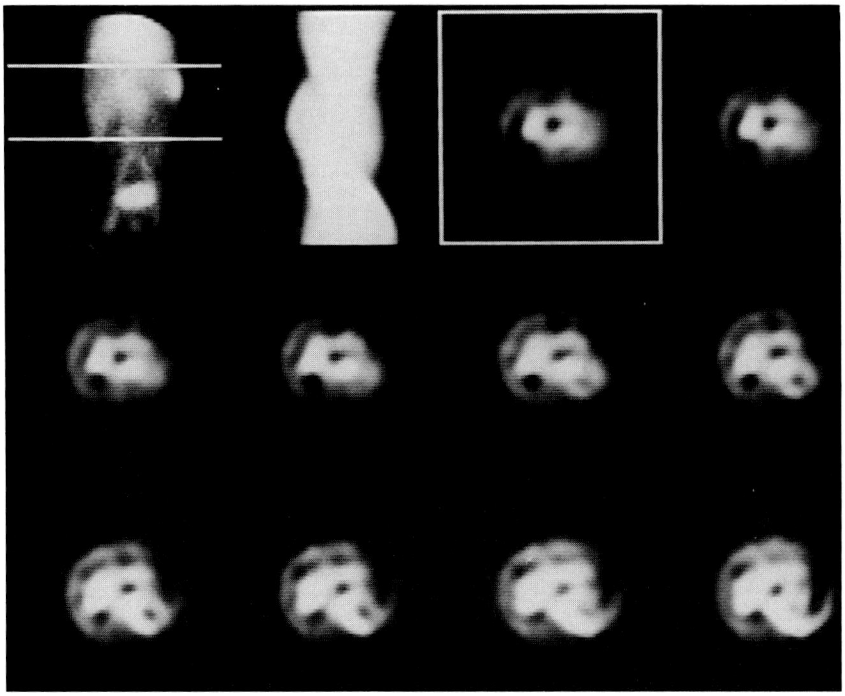

This is a clinical SPECT liver study performed with ^{99m}Tc-labeled red blood cells. A large (>12 mm) uncorrected center-of-rotation error produced dramatic changes in the appearance of the reconstructed transverse sections of the liver. Not only do the images not look anything like a liver, but multiple focal defects are suggested. (The first image in the top row displays the location of the transverse sections that are displayed. The second image is a sinogram that is used for quality control of the data set and evaluating whether the patient moved during the study.) Courtesy of Dr. Mangala Kulkarni.

Comment: These effects from poor center-of-rotation calibration may be seen with any organ imaged. Large errors in center-of-rotation may be easily seen in images of the liver that do not contain focal abnormalities. However, it may be more difficult to identify artifacts from errors of center-of-rotation when imaging nonhomogeneous organs such as lumbar spines or hearts.

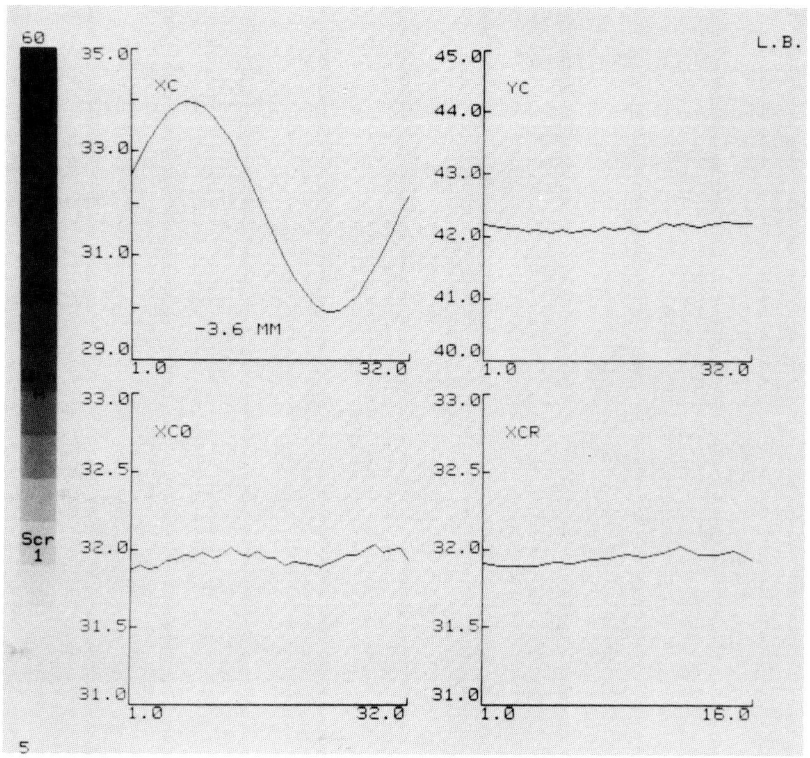

A

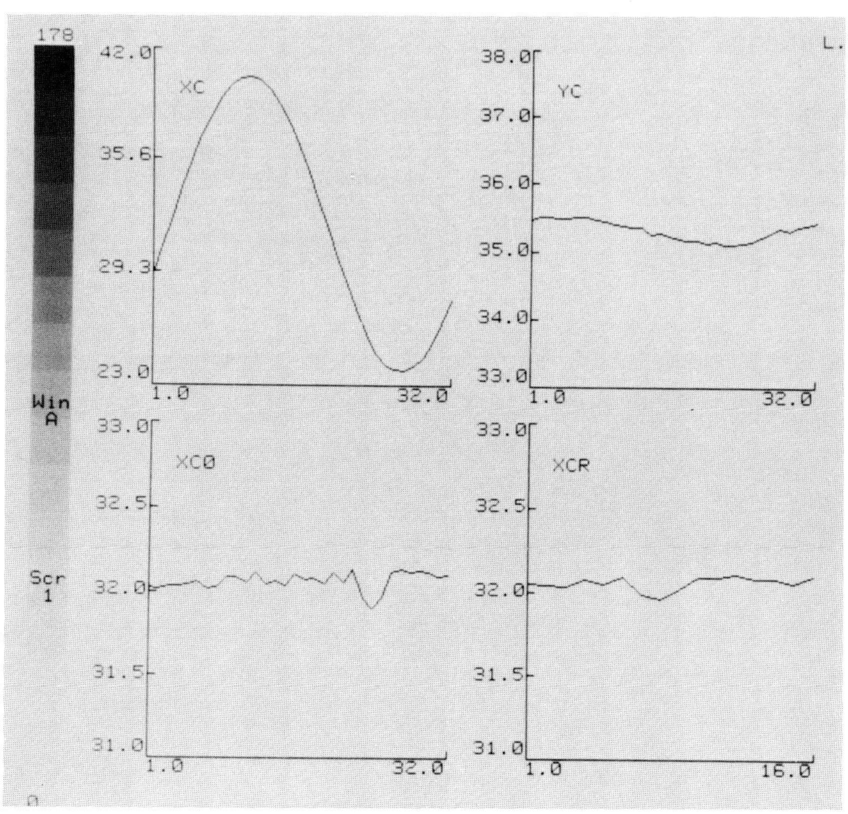

B

Figure 3.3. Center of rotation: analysis of output programs.

The center-of-rotation as a function of the angle of the camera may be obtained by various analysis output programs available from most commerical vendors.

A: Output from General Electric Star II center-of-rotation analysis program. The graph in the upper left shows the fitted sine wave (XC) for the point source calibration data in pixels as a function of gantry angle. The amplitude (y axis) indicates the displacement relative to the center of rotation, and the x axis represents the 32 angles (views). The graph in the lower left (XC0) presents the difference between the fitted sine wave and the actual position in pixels of the centroid of the point source as a function of angle. The graph in the lower right shows the average position of the 16 conjugate pairs (views separated by 180°). The graph in the upper right (YC) indicates the position of the centroid in the Y dimension as a function of angle; that is, it shows if the head is tilted. All parameters are acceptable. The variation in the center of rotation over 32 views (XC0) is less than 0.1 pixel.

Comment: Each individual should become familiar with the center-of-rotation analysis output program for his/her SPECT camera.

B: Output from the same camera as in **A**. Note that in this case the variation in the calibration data over 32 views (XC0) shows a significant positioning error between the 25th and 30th views. Slight bowing of the YC graph indicates the detector was tilted. This would produce a shift of the image in the Y dimension over 360°.

Figure 3.3. continued on following page

(Figure 3.3., cont.)

C: Output of center-of-rotation analysis program shows an average correctable offset error of 0.37 pixel with a standard deviation of 0.174. The maximum acceptable value as stated by the vendor is 0.2. However, the discontinuity in the sinogram reveals incorrect gantry positioning during a segment of data acquisition.

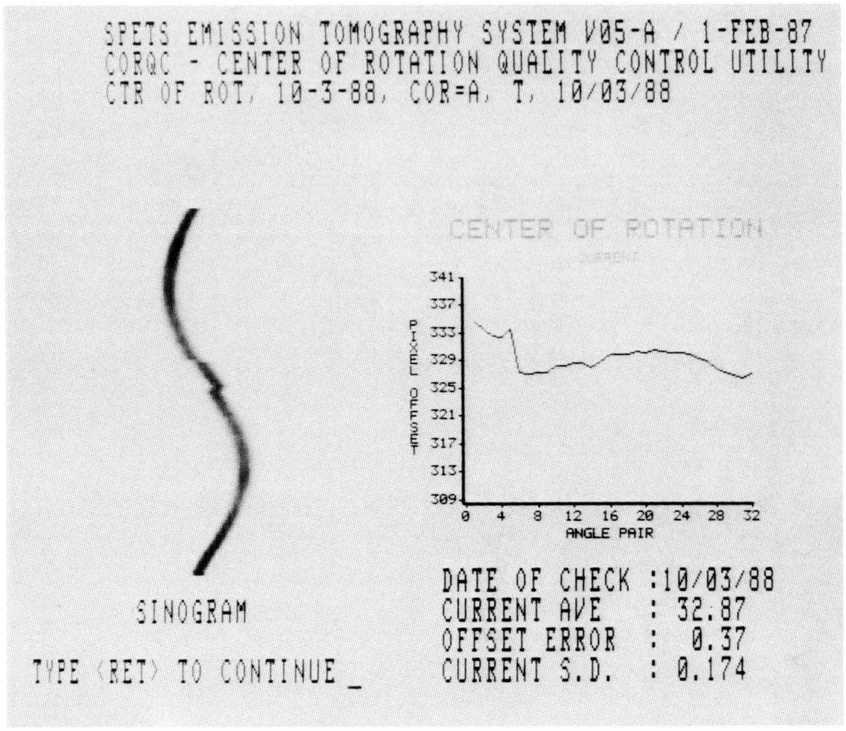

C

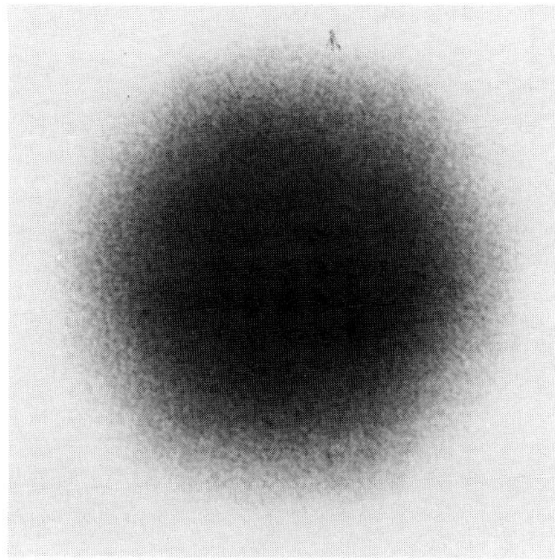

A

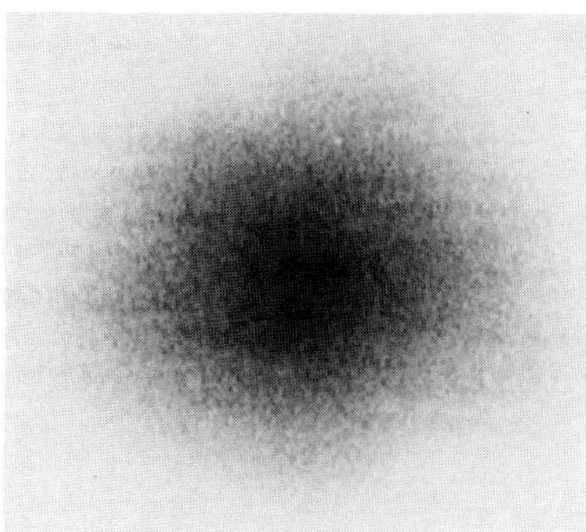

B

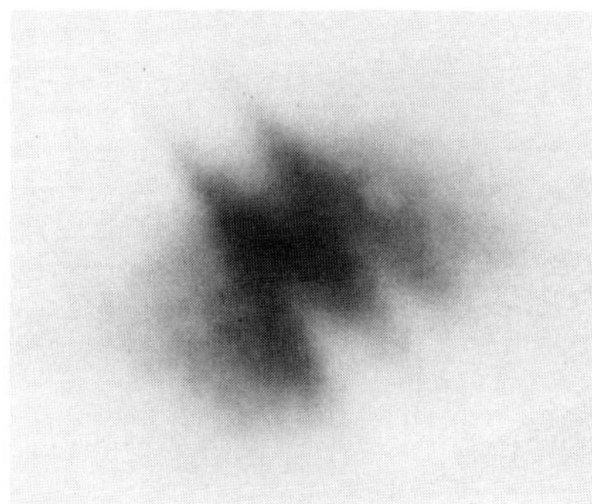

C

Figure 3.4. Parallelism of collimator holes.

Clinical images depend on the holes of the collimator being parallel, and this can be evaluated qualitatively by imaging a distant point source.

A: This image of a point source obtained with a low energy all purpose collimator demonstrates excellent radial symmetry with the intensity decreasing uniformly in all directions from the center to the periphery. This indicates that no significant hole angulation errors are present in the collimator.

B: This image of a point source obtained with a low energy, high resolution collimator shows some hole angulation errors, which is indicated by the presence of striations. These striations are produced when one or more rows of collimator holes are tilted relative to the others. The holes that are "looking" directly at the source will accept more photons than those "looking" off to the side.

Comment: It is unlikely that the magnitude of misalignment seen in this image would have a significant effect on clinical studies; however, ideally all of the holes should be parallel to each other.

C: This image obtained with a low energy general purpose collimator shows marked hole angulation errors.

Comment: This collimator should not be used for clinical SPECT studies.

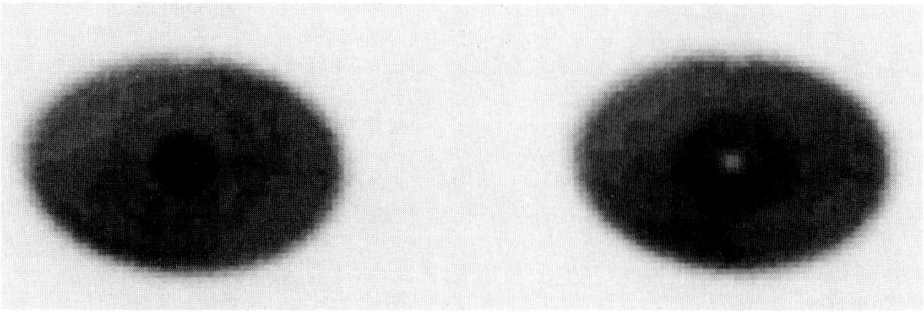

Figure 3.5. Uniformity: quality control.

Two contiguous transverse images of an ellipsoidal phantom containing a uniform solution of $^{99m}TcO_4$ demonstrate "ring" artifacts. Note the marked difference in the appearance of the rings in contiguous slices.
Comment: Good uniformity is very important to help assure good SPECT images. Poor uniformity may result in "ring" artifacts as demonstrated above. The radius of the ring depends on the location of the camera nonuniformity relative to the axis of rotation. The increase or decrease in the apparent activity is determined by the amplitude of the nonuniformity relative to the surrounding area. Crescent artifacts (not shown) are produced when nonuniformity is present in only some of the views.

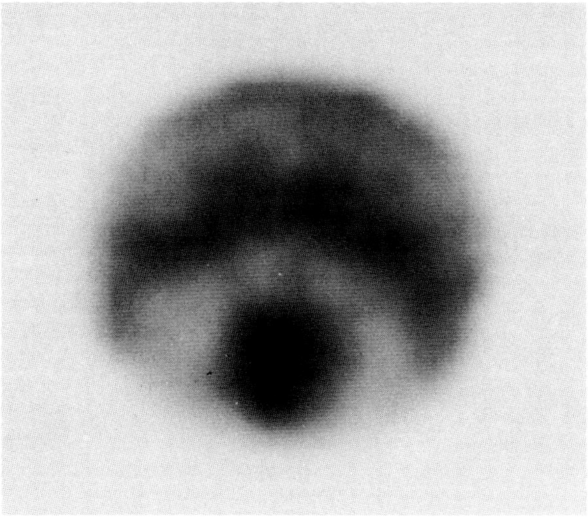

Figure 3.6. Uniformity: quality control.

This is a transverse SPECT image of a Jaszczak phantom, which demonstrates a large ring artifact with a central hot spot due to system nonuniformity (camera and/or collimator). Because the center of the phantom is not on the imaginary line around which the camera rotates (the axis of rotation), the ring appears off-center and semicircular.

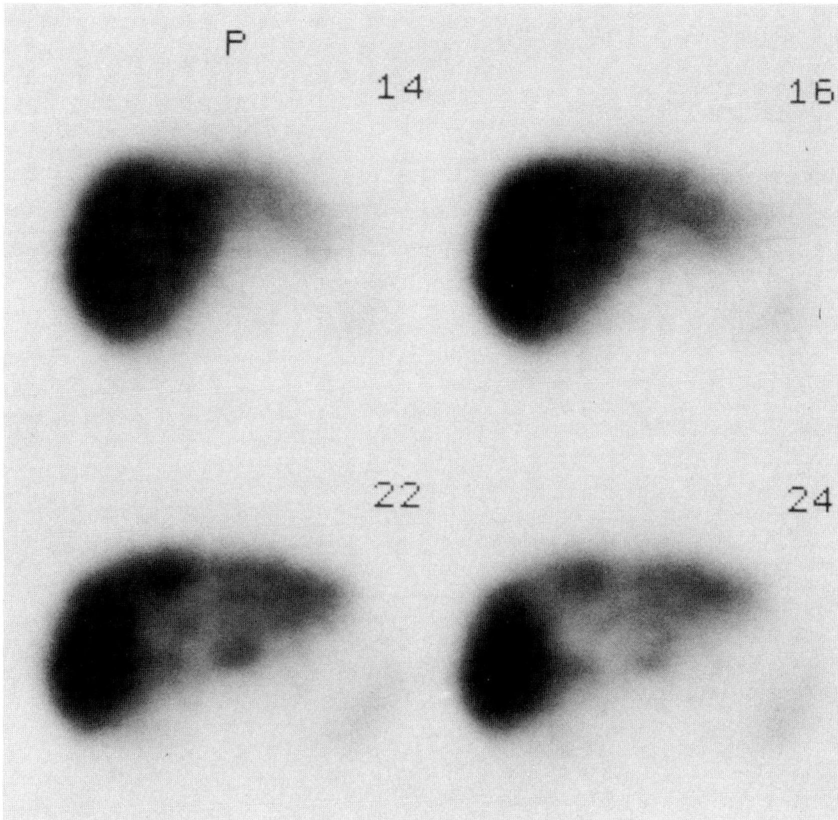

Figure 3.7. Uniformity: clinical examples.

These transverse clinical SPECT images of the liver were obtained with ^{111}In-labeled monoclonal antibodies. Note the ring artifacts present in slices 22 (*lower left*) and 24 (*lower right*).
(Courtesy of Kathleen S. Thomas.)

Figure 3.8. Uniformity: marked nonuniformities.

These images are transverse section images of a Data Spectrum Corporation phantom. Note that in the top row, the intensity of the rings is increased by flood correction. In the bottom row the intensity is decreased, but the ring artifacts are not eliminated.

Comment: Unfortunately, marked nonuniformities in a SPECT system may produce artifacts that are not correctable by high count floods.

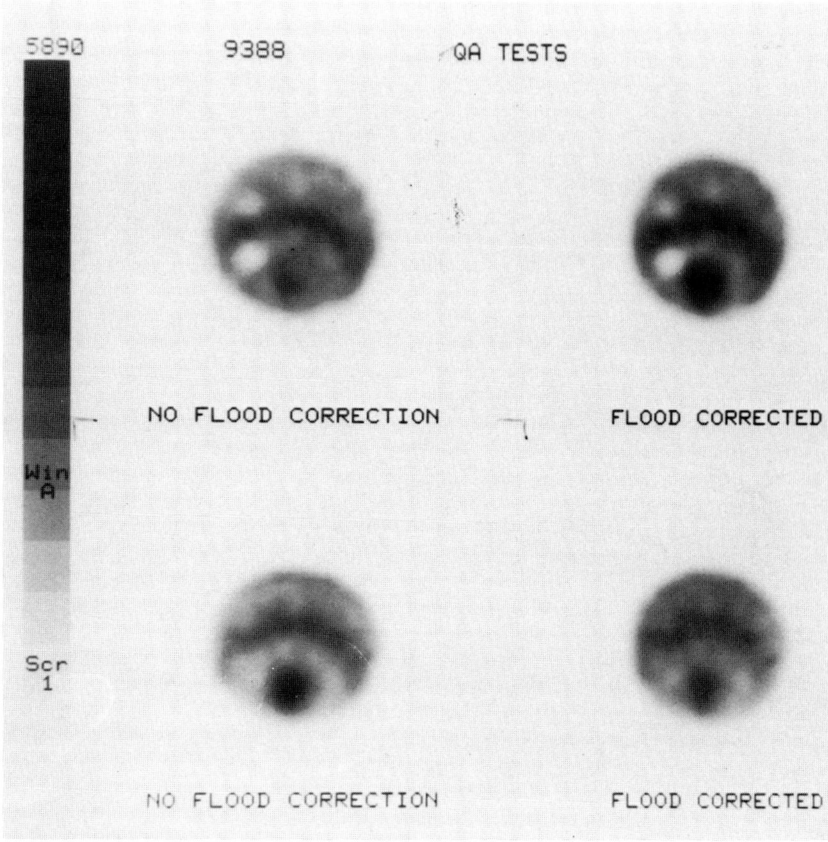

Figure 3.9. Uniformity: miscellaneous.

This is a planar image of a ^{67}Ga point source obtained by a state-of-the-art gamma camera without a light pipe. Note the nonuniform flood, which is most evident in the center of the field of view.

Comment: When imaging such radioisotopes as ^{201}Tl, ^{111}In, or ^{67}Ga, gamma cameras that do not use light pipes typically produce floods and images with more nonuniformity than gamma cameras that use light pipes. Separate intrinsic correction floods may be needed for each radionuclide used to produce artifact-free clinical studies. The visibility of these artifacts is determined by the amplitude of the nonuniformity and the count density of the image.

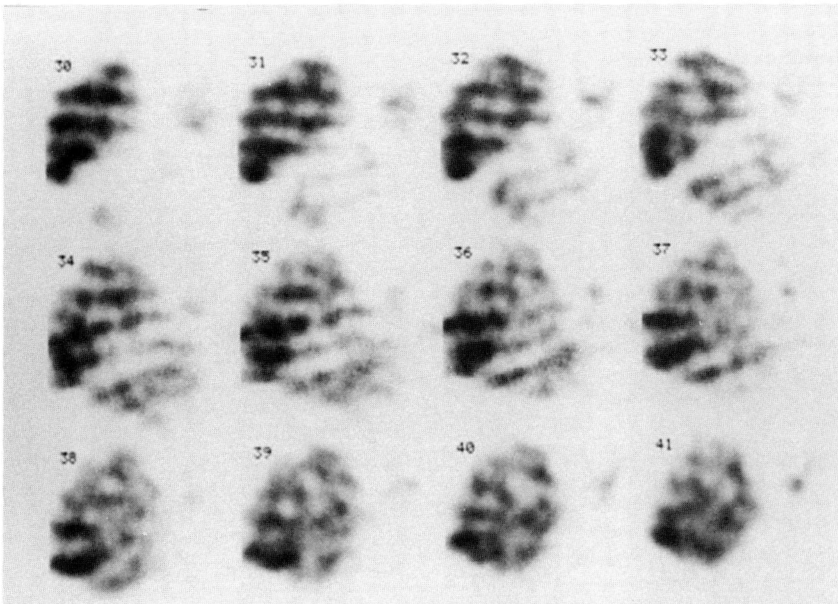

A

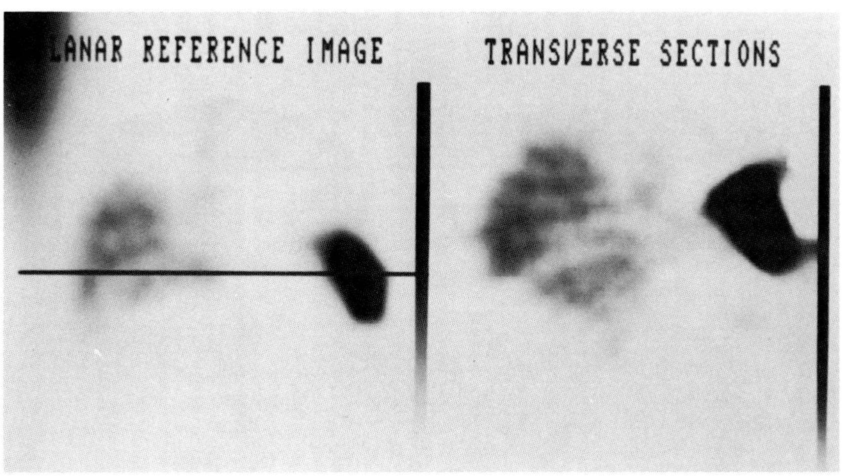

B

Figure 3.10. Streak artifacts.

A: A clinical SPECT study of the liver using the radiopharmaceutical, ^{111}In-labeled leukocytes. Prominent streak artifacts are noted throughout the reconstructed transverse liver (slices 30–41). However, the cause of the streaks is not visible because only the central portion of the image (the liver) is displayed in the reconstructed images.

B: Viewing two of the original images revealed the cause of the streaks. The image on the left is an anterior planar reference image demonstrating marked relatively increased radioactivity in the spleen with significantly less relative activity in the liver. The image on the right is a transverse section with both the liver and spleen in the image. Again, the greater radioactivity in the spleen relative to the liver is clearly apparent.

Comment: Very "hot" sources, in this case the spleen, produce high count streaks when back projection is performed with a limited number of views (e.g., 64). These are superimposed on other parts of the reconstructed image. This problem is inherent in the filtered back projection process and can be reduced only by using more views—128 or 180. Similar artifacts can be produced by a "hot" bladder and extravasation of the injected dose.

(Courtesy of Ellinor Busemann-Sokole.)

Figure 3.11. Phantoms.

A: A "Jaszczak" phantom produced by Data Spectrum Corporation. Models are available with different sphere sizes, circular and ellipsoidal shapes, and various inserts.

Figure 3.11. continued on following page

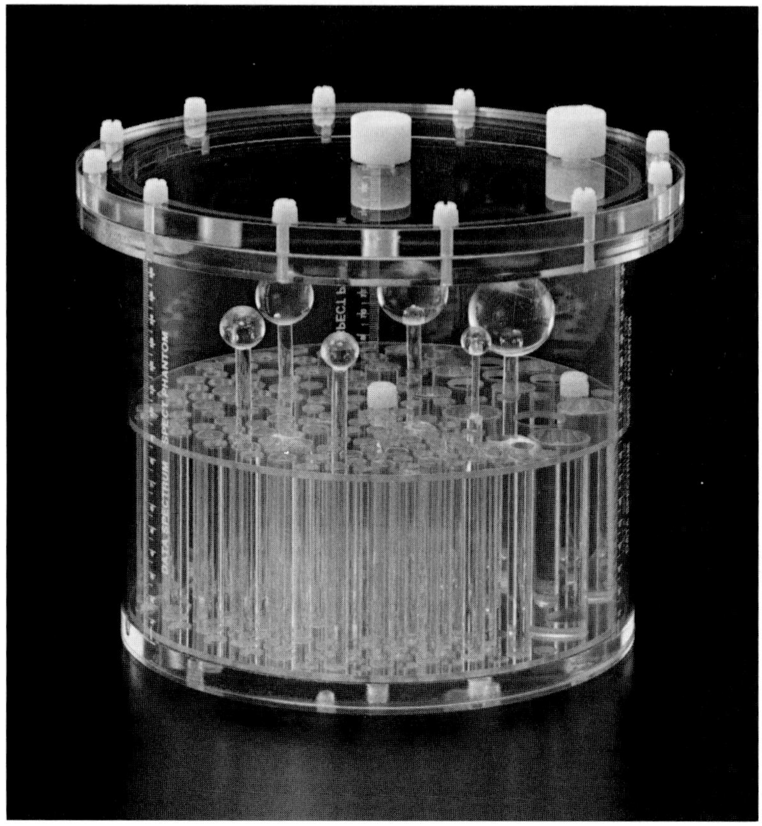

A

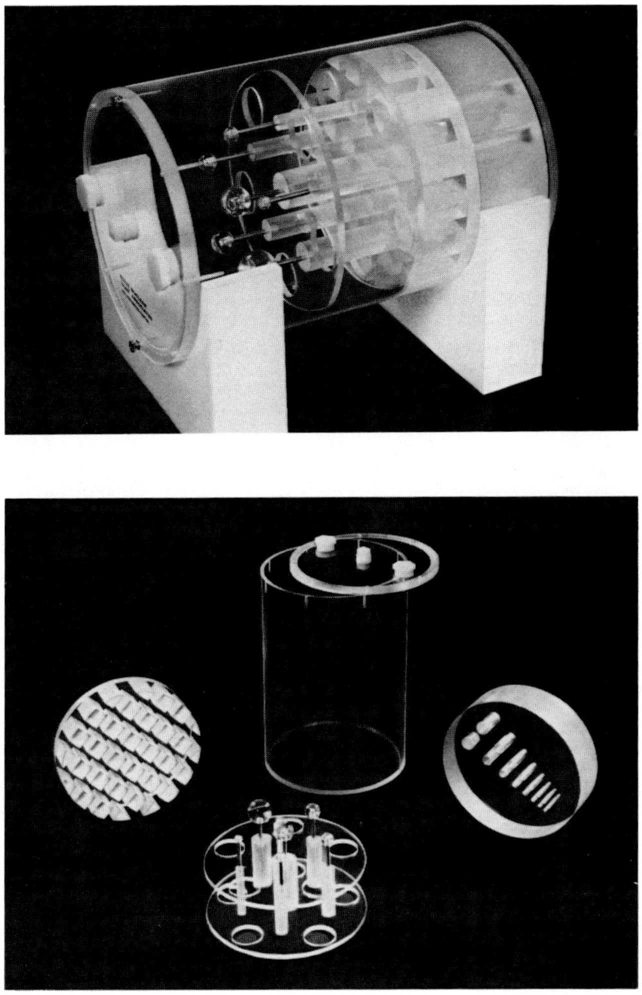

B

(Figure 3.11., cont.)

B: A "Carlson" phantom available from Nuclear Associates. Additional inserts, such as shown in the lower image, can be purchased.
Comment: Phantoms can be useful for quality control of SPECT systems. Each contain a uniform section, a section with cold spheres, and a section that contains a resolution test pattern.

Figure 3.12. Use of phantoms to evaluate attenuation correction.

These images demonstrate the use of the Jaszczak phantom to evaluate attentuation correction, which is one of many parameters that can be evaluated with a phantom. The image on the left in **A** through **D** is the transverse reconstruction of a uniform section of a Jaszczak phantom. The vertical lines down the left image represent a five-pixel wide area that is evaluated for attenuation correction with the corresponding profile curve shown to the right of each image.

A: Without attenuation correction, a vertical profile through the center of the object shows a marked decrease in the center of the image due to absorption of photons.

B: With proper attenuation correction, the same vertical profile is flat except for variations due to statistical fluctuations and reconstruction noise.

C: When the narrow beam attenuation coefficient (0.15/cm) is applied to an image that contains scatter, the profile bulges in the center. This problem can be corrected by using a smaller attenuation coefficient, approximately 0.12/cm.

Figure 3.12. continued on following page

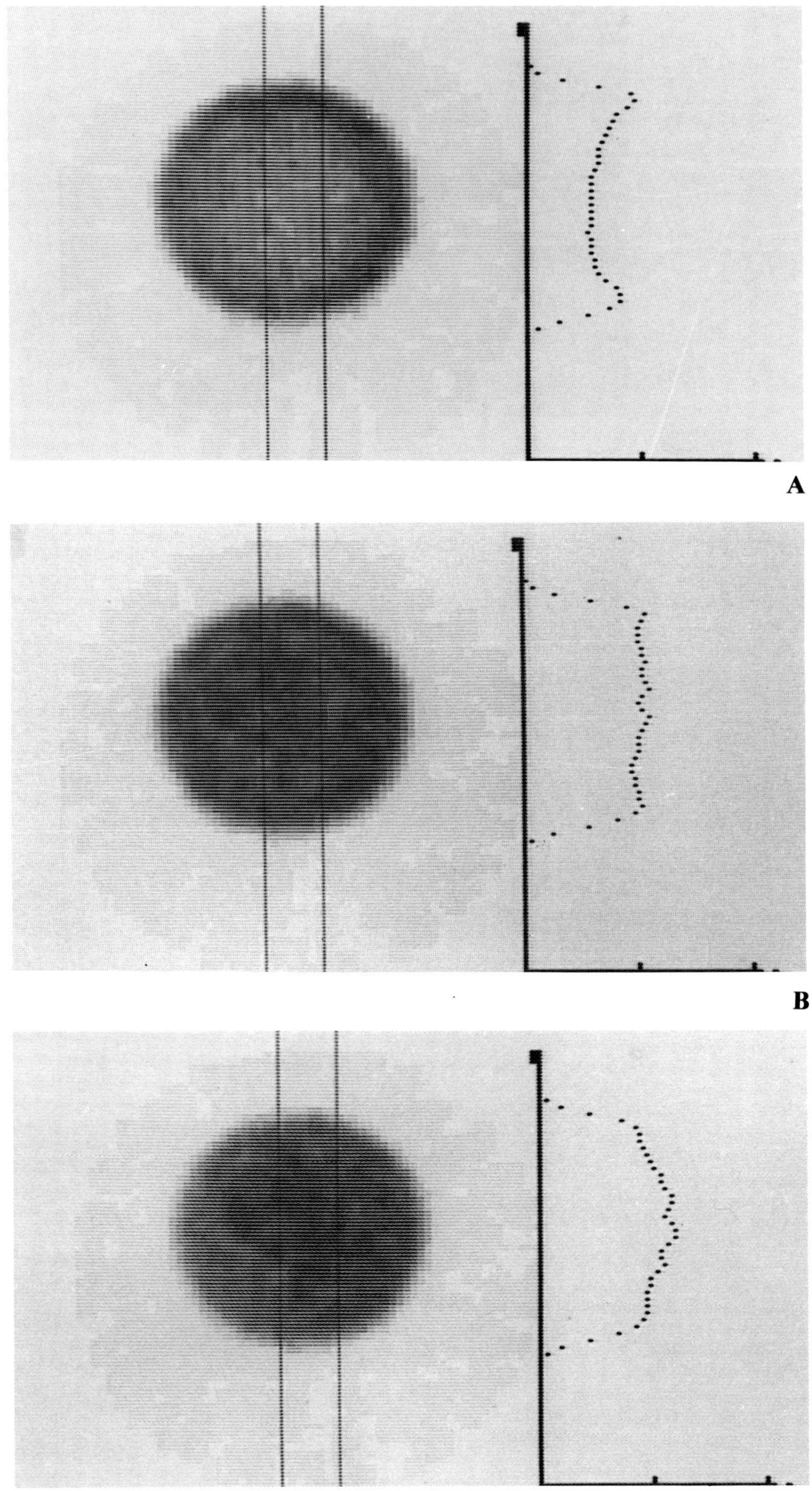

A

B

C

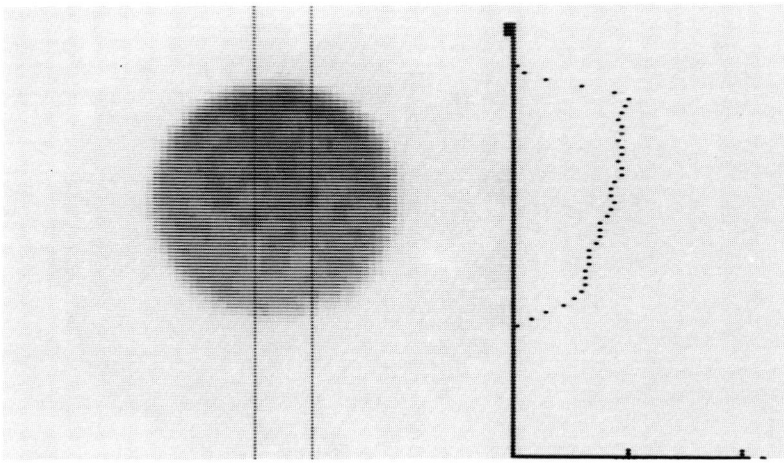

D

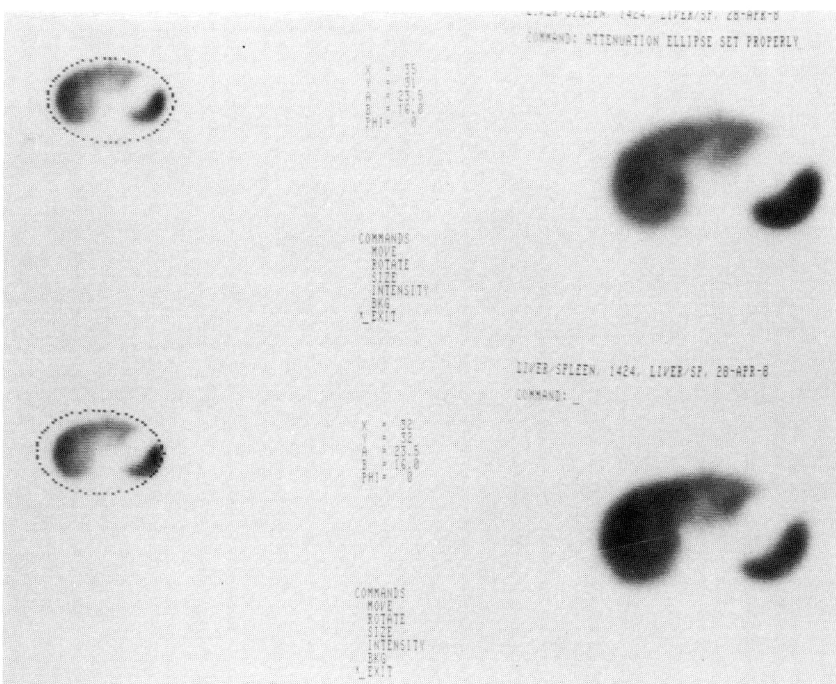

E

(Figure 3.12., cont.)

D: The vertical profile is essentially a straight line when an attenuation coefficient of 0.12/cm is used but it is tilted because the boundaries for attenuation correction were not drawn symmetrically relative to the object. Boundaries should be redrawn and attenuation correction repeated.

E: This clinical SPECT image of the liver demonstrates the change in appearance of the same transverse image of the liver when the boundaries for attenuation correction are not drawn correctly. When the ellipse for attenuation correction (dotted ellipse in left upper compared to left lower image) is shifted to the right, the intensity of the liver in increased and that of the spleen is decreased (right upper compared to right lower image).

Figure 3.13. Use of phantom to evaluate uniformity qualitatively.

A phantom (e.g., Jaszczak) may be used to assess uniformity qualitatively. Eight contiguous transverse slices of a section of a Jaszczak phantom were obtained on an older system that is used for SPECT, and these eight slices are displayed in the first and third rows. Ring artifacts are present. The same eight contiguous transverse slices corrected for uniformity are displayed in the second and fourth rows. One can now assess the ability of the flood correction to correct for the artifacts. In this example, the ring artifacts are significantly reduced.

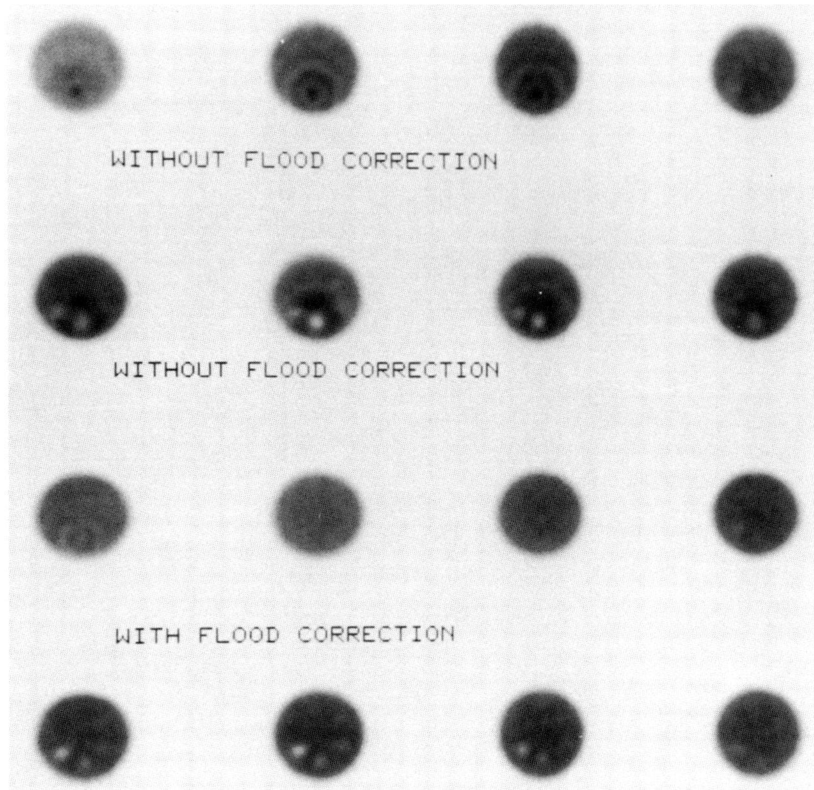

Figure 3.14. Use of phantom to evaluate uniformity quantitatively.

A phantom may be used to assess uniformity quantitatively. A 15 × 15 pixel square ROI is drawn on the center of transverse image obtained from a uniformity SPECT phantom. From this ROI and with the formulas discussed in the text, integral uniformity and noise can be measured.

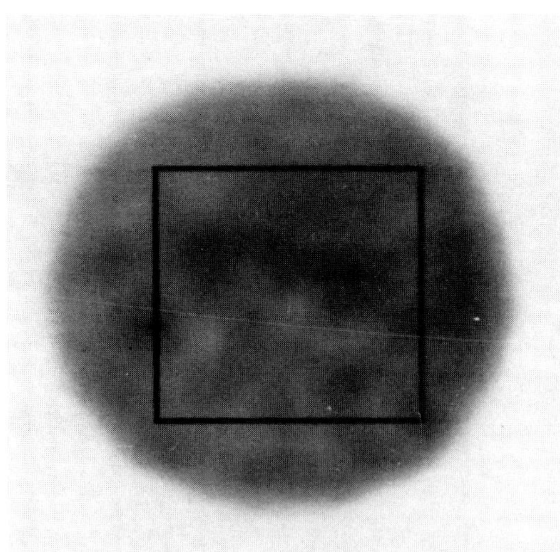

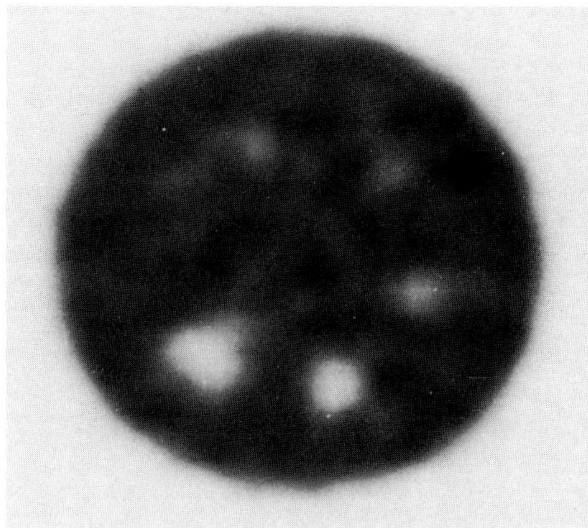

Figure 3.15. Use of phantom to evaluate contrast qualitatively.

A phantom may be used to assess contrast qualitatively. This image is a transverse section of the Jaszczak phantom with solid spheres, which appear "cold" (a Hann filter was used). One may qualitatively assess contrast by noting the number of spheres visualized. For the acquisition and processing conditions listed in Table 3.1, most SPECT systems will show four to five spheres.

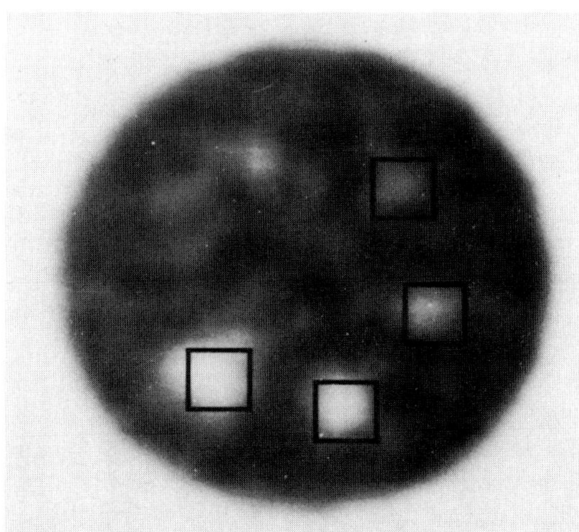

Figure 3.16. Use of phantom to evaluate contrast quantitatively.

A phantom may be used to assess contrast quantitatively. Small ROIs can be drawn on each cold sphere. Statistics from the ROIs often provide the counts in the coolest pixel, which can be used to calculate contrast. See text for details concerning calculation of this parameter.

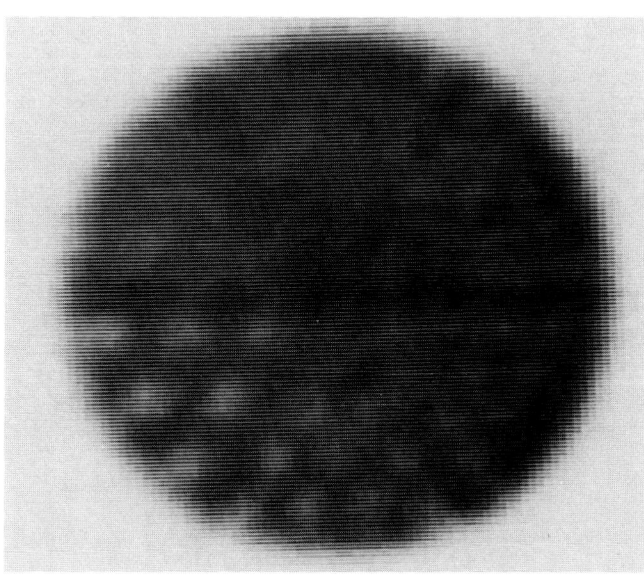

Figure 3.17. Use of phantom to evaluate resolution qualitatively.

This image was produced by the addition of 10 contiguous slices from the lower section of the Data Spectrum Corporation phantom that contains cold rods. This image can be compared to a film obtained at the time of acceptance testing (benchmark film) to evaluate for loss of spatial resolution.

References

1. Keyes JW Jr. Perspectives on tomography. *J Nucl Med*. 1982;23:633–640.
2. Myers MJ, Fazio F. The case for emission computed tomography with a rotating camera. *Appl Radiol/NM*. 1981;10:127–134.
3. Kuhl DE, Barrio JR, Huang SC, et al. Quantifying local cerebral blood flow by N-isopropyl-p[I-123]iodoamphetamine (IMP) tomography. *J Nucl Med*. 1982;23:196–203.
4. Jaszczak RJ, Whitehead FR, Lim CB, et al. Lesion detection with single-photon emission computed tomography (SPECT) compared with conventional imaging. *J Nucl Med*. 1982;23:96–102.
5. Harkness BA, Rogers WL, Clinthorne HN, et al. Quality control procedures and artifact identifications. *J Nucl Med Tech*. 1983;11:55–60.
6. Greer KL, Coleman RE, Jaszczak RJ. SPECT: a practical guide for users. *J Nucl Med Tech*. 1983;11:61–65.
7. English RJ, Brown SE. *SPECT Single-Photon Emission Computed Tomography: A Primer*. New York: The Society of Nuclear Medicine; 1986.
8. Graham LS. A rational quality assurance program for SPECT instrumentation. In: Freeman LM, Weissmann HS, eds. *Nuclear Medicine Annual 1989*. New York: Raven Press; 1989:81–108.
9. Saw CB, Clarke LP, Serafini AN. Influence of zoom factor on centre-of-rotation of the SPECT system and on the resolution of tomographic images. *Nucl Med Commun*. 1987;8:3–12.
10. Single photon emission computerised tomographic (SPECT) systems using rotating scintillation cameras. 1986 draft to be added to Quality Control of Nuclear Medicine Instruments. Vienna: International Atomic Energy Agency; 1984.
11. Chang W, Shuqiang L, Williams JJ, et al. New methods of examining gamma camera collimators. *J Nucl Med*. 1988;29:676–683.
12. Busemann-Sokole E. Measurement of collimator hole angulation and camera head tilt for slant and parallel hole collimators used in SPECT. *J Nucl Med*. 1987;28:1592–1598.
13. Malmin RE, Stanley PC, Guth WR. Collimator angulation error and its effect on SPECT. *J Nucl Med*. 1990;31:655–659.
14. Silverstein EA, Spies SM. Evaluation of parallel hole collimators used for SPECT imaging. *Phys Med Biol*. 1988;33(Suppl I):112. Abstract
15. Lamoureux G, Verba J, Halpern SE. A new technique for the evaluation of hole parallelism in collimators used for SPECT. *Clin Nucl Med*. 1988; 13(Suppl):P20.
16. Rogers WL, Clinthorne HN, Harkness BA, et al. Flood-field requirements for emission computed tomography with an Anger camera. *J Nucl Med*. 1982;23:162–168.
17. Todd-Pokropek A, Zerowski S, Soussaline F. Nonuniformity and artifact creation in emission tomography. *J Nucl Med*. 1980;21:P38. Abstract.
18. Collier BD, Slizofski WJ, Krasnow AZ. SPECT bone imaging (lumbar spine, hips, knees, and temporomandibular joint). In: Van Nostrand D, Baum S, eds. *Atlas of Nuclear Medicine*. Philadelphia: JB Lippincott Co; 1988:360–382.
19. Burst KD, Graham MM. Aspects of patient imaging with SPECT. *J Nucl Med*. 1987;15:133–137.

CHAPTER 4

Atlas of Normal Bone Scan and ^{111}In White Blood Cell Findings in Porous-Coated Hip Prostheses

Stephen G. Oswald and Douglas Van Nostrand

The nuclear medicine physician is often asked to evaluate the patient with a painful hip prosthesis with specific regard to the presence of loosening or infection. The scintigraphic findings for complicated and uncomplicated cemented hip prostheses have been well described.[1-4] Recently, hip arthroplasty using porous-coated protheses has gained popularity. Since prosthesis fixation occurs as bone and fibrous tissue grow into the porous surface of the prosthesis,[5] increased localization of bone-avid isotopes might occur unrelated to the presence of aseptic loosening or infection. It is necessary to know the scintigraphic appearance of the uncomplicated porous-coated prosthesis to diagnose reliably the presence of an abnormality.

This atlas demonstrates the spectrum of three-phase bone (TPBS) and ^{111}In-labeled white blood cell (In-WBC) scintigraphy in patients with uncomplicated porous-coated hip arthroplasties (PCHA). It contains examples previously published in the *Journal of Nuclear Medicine*[6,7] as well as additional images and graphs that have not been published. The data are derived from our analysis of 25 uncomplicated porous-coated prostheses in 21 patients followed prospectively with serial TPBS and In-WBC over a 2-year period. The TPBS and In-WBC scans were obtained at approximately 7 days and at 3, 6, 12, 18, and 24 months postoperatively. No patient developed aseptic loosening or infection of the prosthesis during the study. This atlas allows us to bring together all the images in a single publication and to present additional material, providing examples of the natural history of scintigraphic changes in this population. We hope this atlas will be helpful in interpreting TPBS or In-WBC in patients with PCHA.

Technique

Imaging Procedure: Bone Scintigraphy

Flow Study

Twenty mCi (740 MBq) of ^{99m}Tc methylene diphosphonate (Tc-MDP) were injected into the antecubital vein using a bolus injection technique. Serial anterior images were acquired over the hip and proximal femur every 3 to 4 sec for 30 sec.

Blood Pool

An anterior image was obtained over the prosthesis approximately 5 min after radionuclide injection. The image was acquired for 750,000 to 1 million counts for small and large field of view cameras, respectively.

Bone Phase

The bone phase images over the anterior hip were acquired 2.5 to 3 hr after injection for 750,000 to 1 million counts, depending on the type of gamma camera. A low energy general purpose collimator was used. Images were graded by comparing activity in the area of interest with the ipsilateral iliac crest. This is easily done by obtaining an image that encompasses the iliac crest and the prosthesis tip in the same field of view. If a second image is required to visualize the entire area, it should be acquired for the same length of time as the first image.

In-WBC Scintigraphy

Labeling of WBC was performed according to standard technique[8] and 500 μCi (18.5 MBq) of ^{111}In-labeled WBCs were reinjected into the patient. Images were acquired 18 to 24 hr later with a medium energy collimator using a 20% window centered about the 245-KeV energy peak and a 15% window asymmetrically placed about the 172-KeV peak. This method allowed us to perform TPBS and In-WBC on consecutive days without significant interference between ^{99m}Tc and ^{111}In energy peaks. An alternate acquisition method to assure that any residual ^{99m}Tc activity will not be inadvertently detected in a window set for the lower ^{111}In energy peak (172 KeV) involves acquisition using only the 245-KeV ^{111}In energy peak. Images were obtained for 200,000 to 500,000 for small to large field of view cameras.

Grading of Activity

Flow and Blood Pool

The flow and blood pool images were graded by comparing activity in the area of interest with activity in the contralateral iliac vessel. Intensity of activity greater than soft tissue background but less than iliac vessel was considered 1+, equal to iliac vessel was 2+, and activity was 3+ if greater than iliac intensity.

Bone Phase and In-WBC

The bone and In-WBC images were compared to the ipsilateral iliac crest. Activity less than iliac crest but greater than background (defined as uptake in a normal adjacent or contralateral bone area) was graded as 1+, equal to iliac crest was graded as 2+, and greater than iliac crest was regarded as 3+. Care should be taken that the patient is lying flat on the imaging table and not slightly turned or rotated. This assures that the prosthesis and the iliac crest remain at constant distances from the camera face on serial scans.

Computer Acquisition

None.

Estimated Absorbed Radiation Dose

Bone Scintigraphy

Absorbed radiation dose (adapted from product literature insert, MPI MDP Kit, Medi-Physics, Inc., Paramus, NJ).

Organ	rad/20 mCi	mGy/740 MBq
Total body	0.13	1.3
Bone total	0.70	7.0
Red marrow	0.56	5.6
Kidneys	0.80	8.0
Liver	0.06	0.6
Bladder wall		
2-hr void	2.60	26.0
4.8-hr void	6.20	62.0
Ovaries		
2-hr void	0.24	2.4
4.8-hr void	0.34	3.4
Testes		
2-hr void	0.16	1.6
4.8-hr void	0.22	2.2

In-WBC Scintigraphy

Absorbed radiation dose (adapted from product literature insert, ^{111}In oxine, Amersham Corporation, Arlington Heights, IL).

Organ	rad/500 μCi	mGy/18.5 MBq
Spleen	13	130
Liver	1.9	19
Red marrow	1.3	13
Skeleton	0.364	3.64
Testes	0.01	0.1
Ovaries	0.19	1.9
Total body	0.31	3.1

Visual Description and Interpretation

Ideally, the images should be approached initially without the benefit of clinical information. Flow, blood pool, bone, and/or In-WBC images should be evaluated for presence of activity about the prosthesis, as well as the intensity, pattern, and location of activity. Comparison should be made with any previous scan for change in intensity, pattern, and location of activity. Radiographs ideally should be present for comparison. The initial impression should be reevaluated in light of the pertinent clinical history, such as the time of surgery, type of prosthesis, and site of pain. A brief interview with the patient regarding character and location of pain may be helpful. If the In-WBC study is acquired in close proximity to the TPBS, images must be evaluated for possible inappropriate setting of acquisition energy windows, resulting in visualization of activity from residual ^{99m}Tc, and potentially causing a false positive study.

The following atlas discusses the findings in a series of uncomplicated, uncemented (porous-coated) hip prostheses and should provide an initial data base for interpretation of images related to these prostheses. Since no prosthesis became loose or infected during the 24-month evaluation period, no analysis of sensitivity or specificity in diagnosing these entities is possible. Our data differ somewhat from that which has been previously reported for cemented prostheses.[4] It is our belief that knowing the type of prosthesis (cemented vs. uncemented) is important for proper interpretation of TPBS or In-WBC as it relates to hip arthroplasty.

Atlas Section

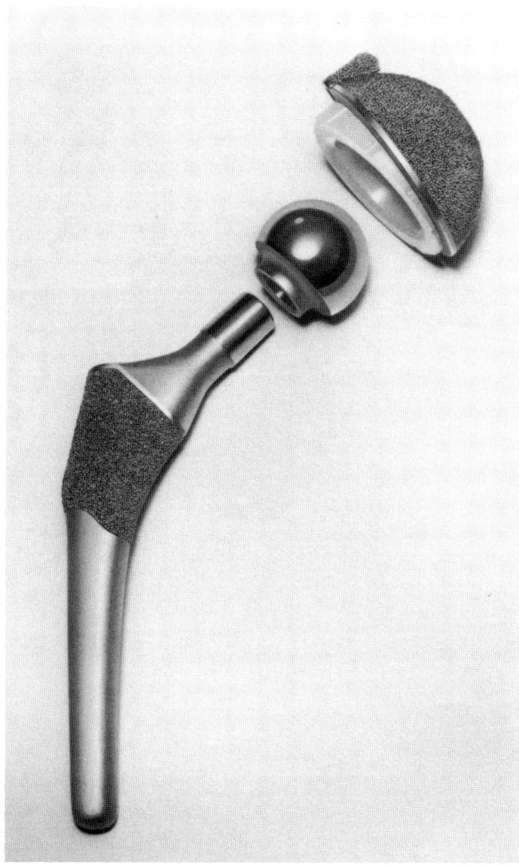

General

Figure 4.1. An example of the porous-coated prosthesis (PCA Total Hip System) used in our study.

(Photo provided courtesy of Howmedica, Inc., Division of Pfizer Hospital Products Group, Inc.)

Figure 4.2. Schematic diagram of a porous-coated prosthesis.

This diagram identifies the various regions of the prosthesis discussed below. ACE, acetabulum; GT, greater trochanter; LT, lesser trochanter; TIP, prosthesis tip. The tip is further subdivided as follows: MS, medial tip segment; DS, distal tip segment; LS, lateral tip segment. The stippling represents the porous-coated area.

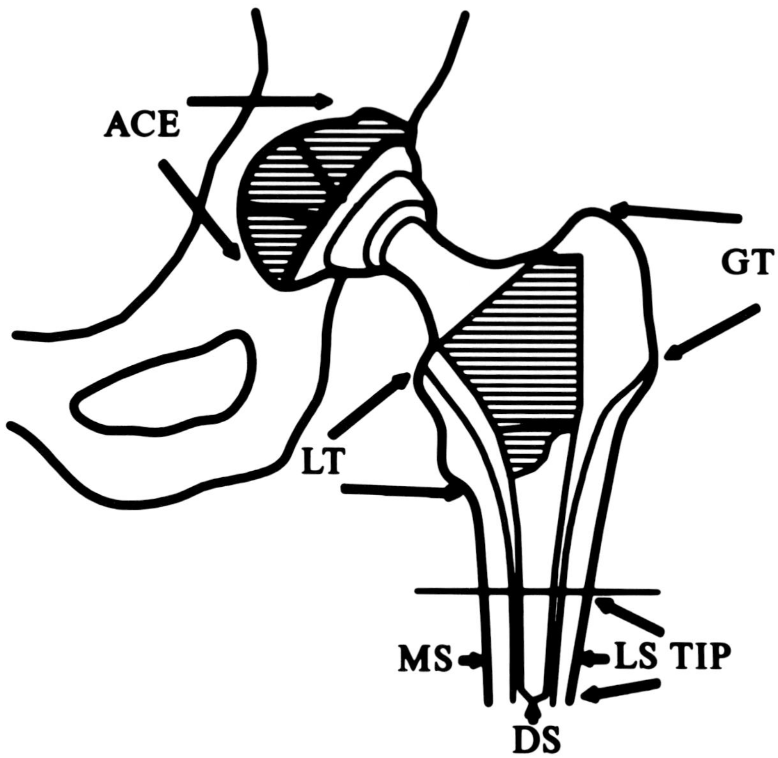

Three-Phase Bone Scan

Tip

Flow Study

Figure 4.3. Normal blood flow study of prosthesis tip.

Sequential anterior images over the hip demonstrate normal blood flow in the vicinity of the prosthesis tip. Skin markers (*arrows*) indicate greater trochanters.
Comment: External markers are recommended to help with orientation on flow and blood pool images.

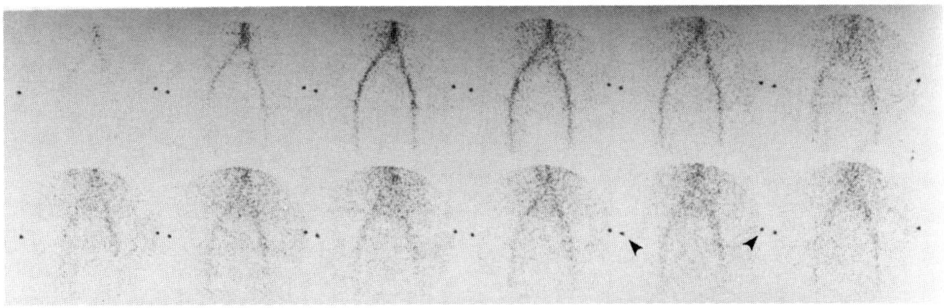

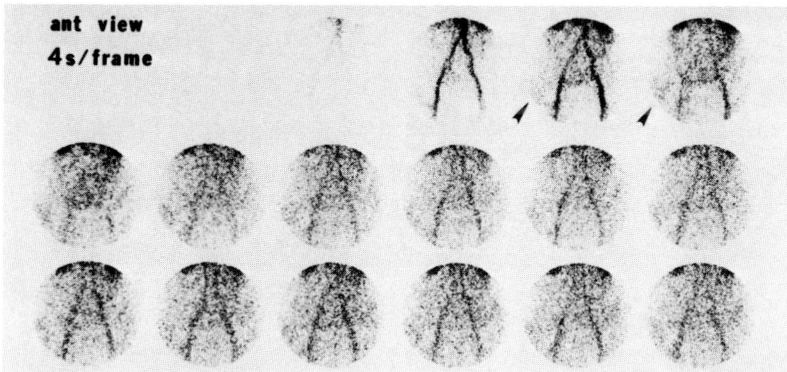

Figure 4.4. Increased blood flow at prosthesis tip.

Mildly increased flow was noted (*arrows*) on the 7-day scan in this patient.

Comment: Increased blood flow to the region of the prosthesis tip is an unusual finding in the uncomplicated PCHA, noted in only 1 of 136 scans. Increased blood flow at the prosthesis tip should raise the suspicion that a complication is present.

Blood Pool

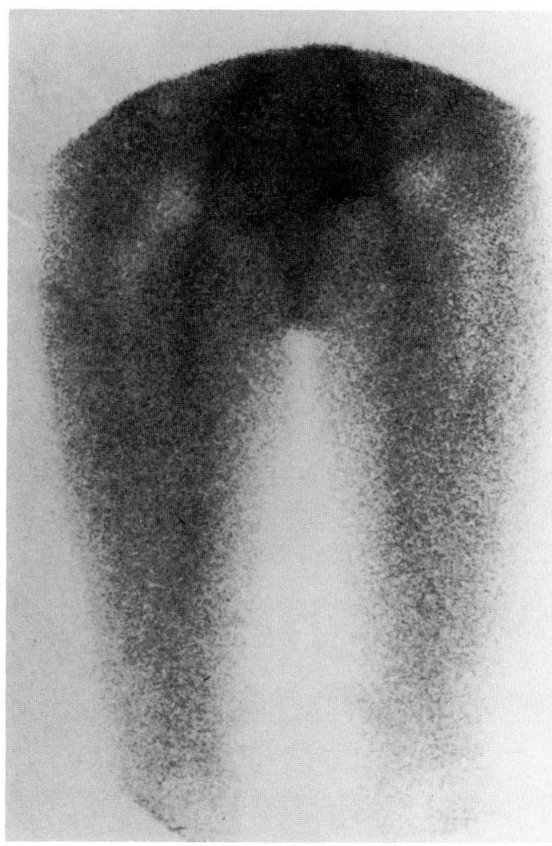

Figure 4.5. Normal blood pool of prosthesis tip.

Anterior image demonstrates no increased activity at the tips of bilateral prostheses. A photon deficiency due to attenuation by the prosthesis is noted bilaterally.

Figure 4.6. Focally increased blood pool at prosthesis tip.

Minimally increased activity (*arrows*) is seen in the blood pool images of two patients. *Bottom row:* blood pool image. *Top row:* corresponding bone phase image shown for orientation. Note the subtle asymmetry of activity between the side with the prosthesis and the normal femur. See Comment of Fig. 4.7.

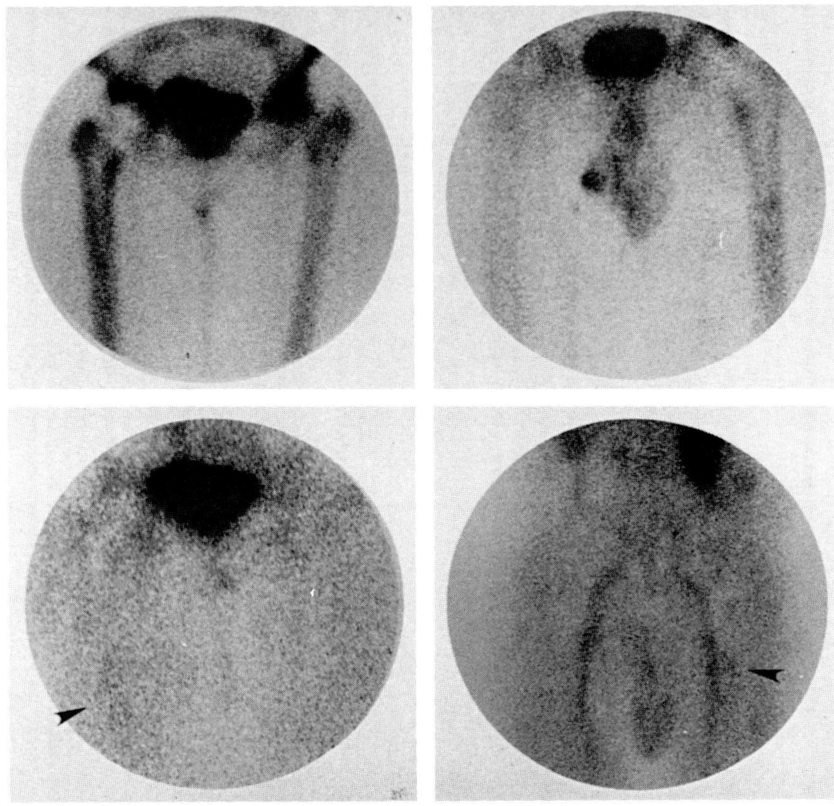

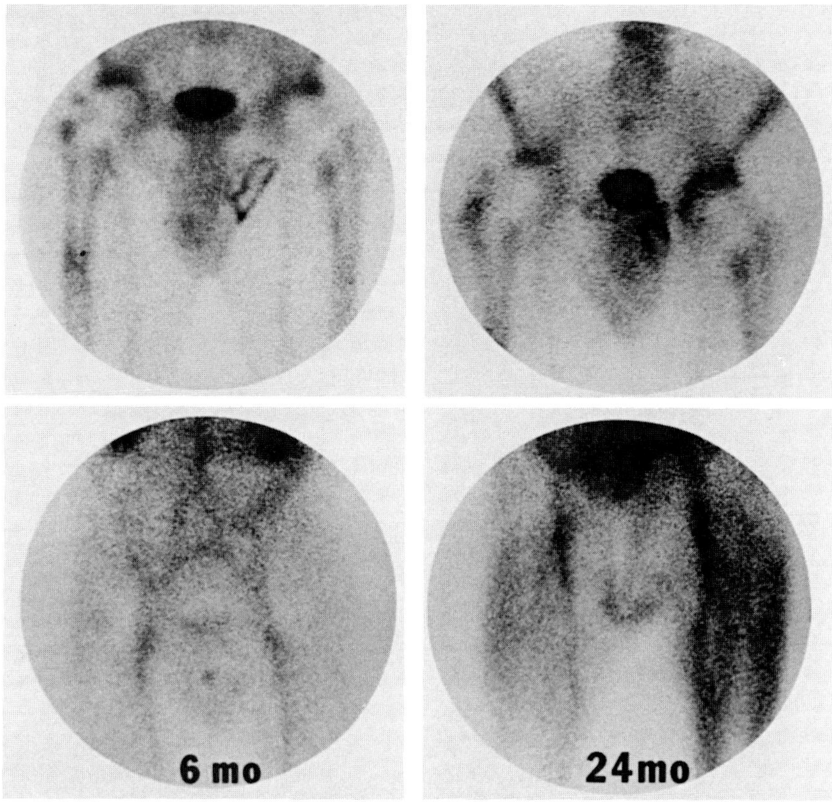

Figure 4.7. Diffusely increased blood pool of thigh.

The blood pool images (*bottom row*) demonstrate the development of diffusely increased activity throughout the left thigh in a patient with bilateral prostheses. *Top row:* corresponding bone phase images shown for orientation.

Comment: There were two types of increased blood pool activity noted—focal and diffuse. Focally increased activity at the prosthesis tip was an unusual finding, appearing in only 2 of 136 scans in our patient population, at 3 and 6 months after arthroplasty, respectively. Therefore, the presence of focal blood pool activity should probably be viewed with suspicion. The diffusely increased activity noted throughout the thigh was seen in 20 of 136 scans (11 of the 25 prostheses) but was never seen before 12 months postoperatively. The etiology of this activity is uncertain but this diffuse activity is unlikely to represent a complication. We speculate that this may be due to increased muscle usage.

(Reprinted with permission from the *Journal of Nuclear Medicine*; 1989;30:1321–1331; The Society of Nuclear Medicine.)

Bone Phase

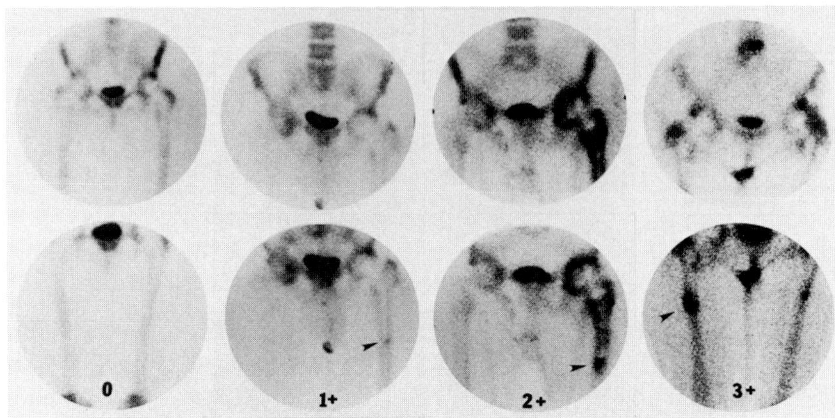

Figure 4.8. Examples of intensity grades of tip uptake.

Bottom row: The spectrum of intensity of Tc-MDP uptake at the tip. Grade 0 represented no activity above normal background (defined as uptake in normal femur), grade 1+ was activity greater than background but less than iliac crest, grade 2+ was equal to ipsilateral iliac crest, and grade 3+ was greater than iliac crest. Images of the pelvis for each patient are shown in the top row so that comparison can be made with the iliac crest. The pelvic images were obtained on the same camera for the same length of time and at the same photographic intensity as the images of the prosthesis tip.
Comment: Tc-MDP uptake at the tip was found in 120 of 143 scans and in all 25 prostheses at some time during the 24 months of postoperative observation. The presence of increased activity on bone scan alone does not predict the presence of loosening or infection.
(Reprinted with permission from the *Journal of Nuclear Medicine*; 1989;30:1321–1331; The Society of Nuclear Medicine.)

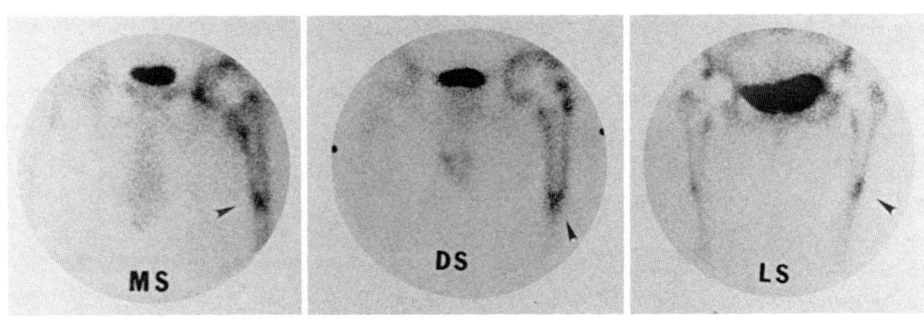

Figure 4.9. Preferential localization of tip activity.

When tip uptake was stratified as to its precise location, Tc-MDP uptake (*arrowheads*) often predominated in one or more of the tip subdivisions. MS, scan showing preferential localization in the medial tip segment; DS, localization in the distal segment; LS, localization in the lateral segment.
Comment: A comparison of activity grades between tip segments for each image indicated that intensity of uptake in the MS was less than LS intensity in 30% of scans, equal to LS intensity in 69% of scans, and greater than LS in only 1% of scans. Since medial segment intensity greater than lateral segment was a rare finding, it should be viewed with suspicion.
(Reprinted with permission from the *Journal of Nuclear Medicine*; 1989;30:1321–1331; The Society of Nuclear Medicine.)

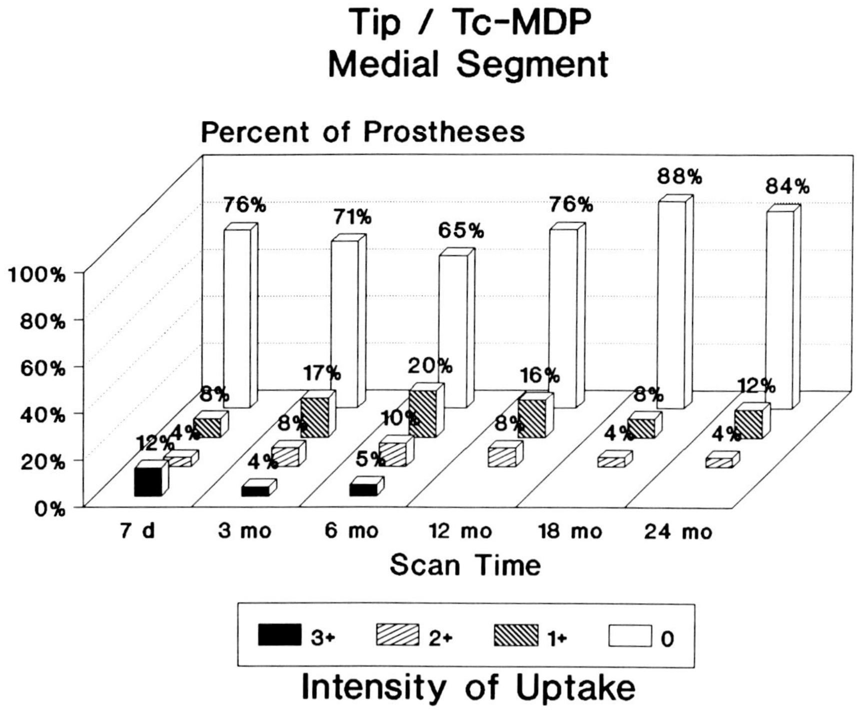

Figure 4.10. Medial segment activity.

The graph demonstrates the percentage of prostheses exhibiting a given intensity of Tc-MDP uptake in the medial segment of the prosthesis tip at the various scanning times. See Comment in Fig. 4.11.
(Reprinted with permission from the *Journal of Nuclear Medicine*; 1989;30:1321–1331; The Society of Nuclear Medicine.)

Figure 4.11. Trend in medial segment activity.

The percentage of prostheses exhibiting a particular trend in changing medial segment Tc-MDP intensity during a given time interval. For example, for the interval encompassing the 6th through 24th month postoperatively, 88% of prostheses had stable or decreasing activity, 12% exhibited an increase in intensity by 1 grade at some point during this time interval, and none showed an increase by two or more grades. **Comment:** The majority of prostheses demonstrate grade 0 activity in the medial segment. Activity greater than or equal to the iliac crest (2+ and 3+) becomes less frequent with time. Given the predilection for decreasing medial segment activity with time, any increasing activity within the medial segment, especially after the first few months postoperatively, should be viewed with suspicion. Comparison with a baseline scan can be particularly helpful and strong consideration should be given to obtaining such a study. As an alternative to obtaining baseline scans in all patients, only those who develop pain could be scanned. This would become the baseline examination with a repeat scan and clinical evaluation performed in 3 months.

(Reprinted with permission from the *Journal of Nuclear Medicine*; 1989;30:1321–1331; The Society of Nuclear Medicine.)

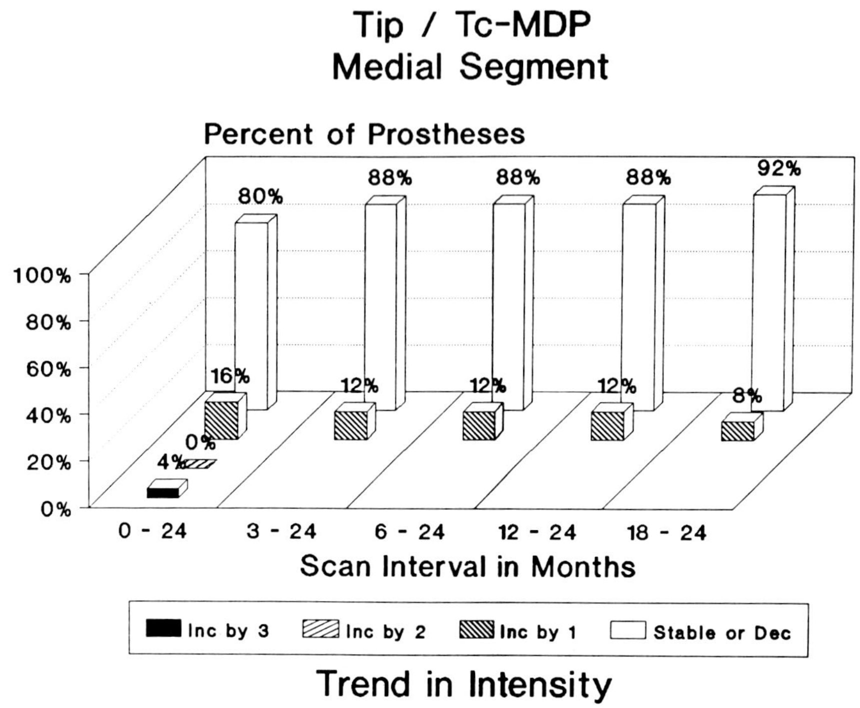

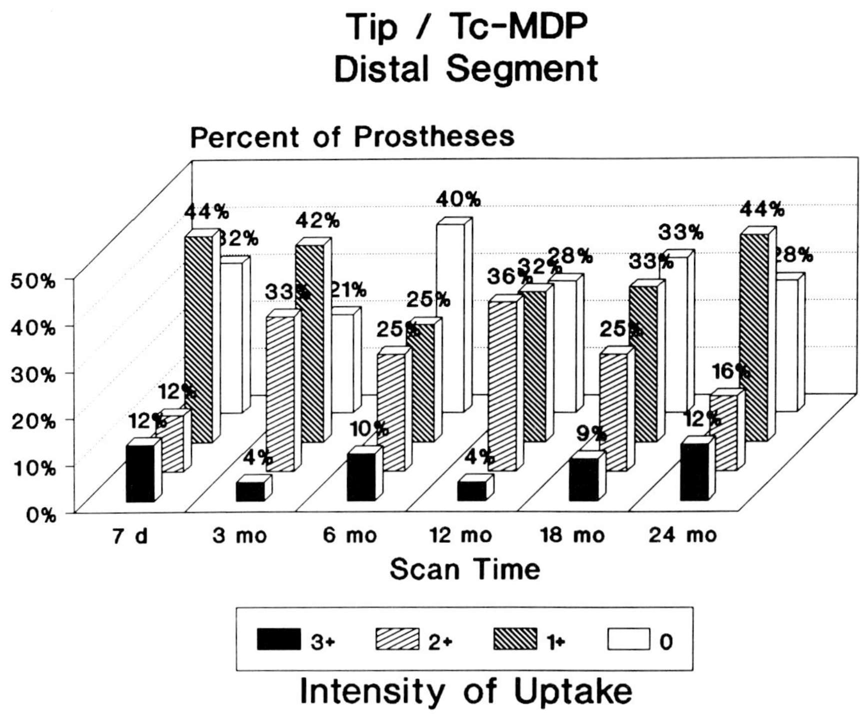

Figure 4.12. Distal segment activity.

The percentage of prostheses with a particular grade of distal segment uptake at a given scanning time. See Comment in Fig. 4.13. (Reprinted with permission from the *Journal of Nuclear Medicine*; 1989;30:1321–1331; The Society of Nuclear Medicine.)

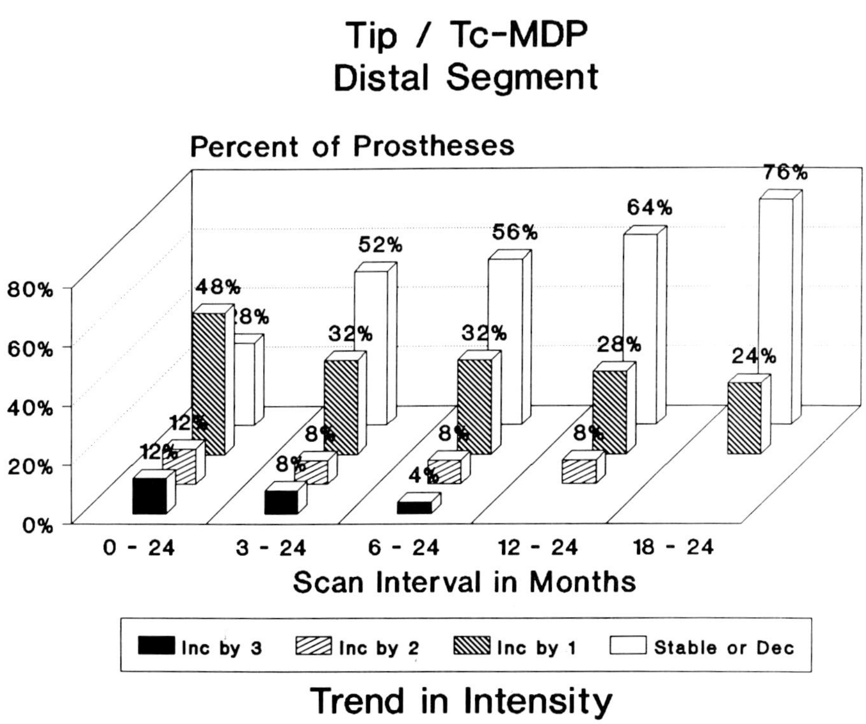

Figure 4.13. Trend in distal segment activity.

The percentage of prostheses exhibiting a particular trend in changing distal segment Tc-MDP intensity during a given time interval. For example, during the time interval encompassing 6 to 24 months postoperatively, 56% of prostheses showed stable or decreasing activity, in 32% activity increased by one intensity grade, and in 8% and 4% activity increased by two and three intensity grades, respectively.

Comment: Although a considerable percentage of prostheses have significant activity remaining at the distal tip segment at 24 months postoperatively, the trend over serial scans is for activity to remain stable or decline. This presence of focal uptake alone does not necessarily signify a complication. However, increasing activity over time should be viewed with suspicion. In addition, the greater and the later the increase, the greater the suspicion.

(Reprinted with permission from the *Journal of Nuclear Medicine*; 1989;30:1321–1331; The Society of Nuclear Medicine.)

Figure 4.14. Lateral segment activity.

The percentage of prostheses exhibiting a given intensity of Tc-MDP uptake at the various scanning times. See Comment in Fig. 4.15.
(Reprinted with permission from the *Journal of Nuclear Medicine*; 1989;30:1321–1331; The Society of Nuclear Medicine.)

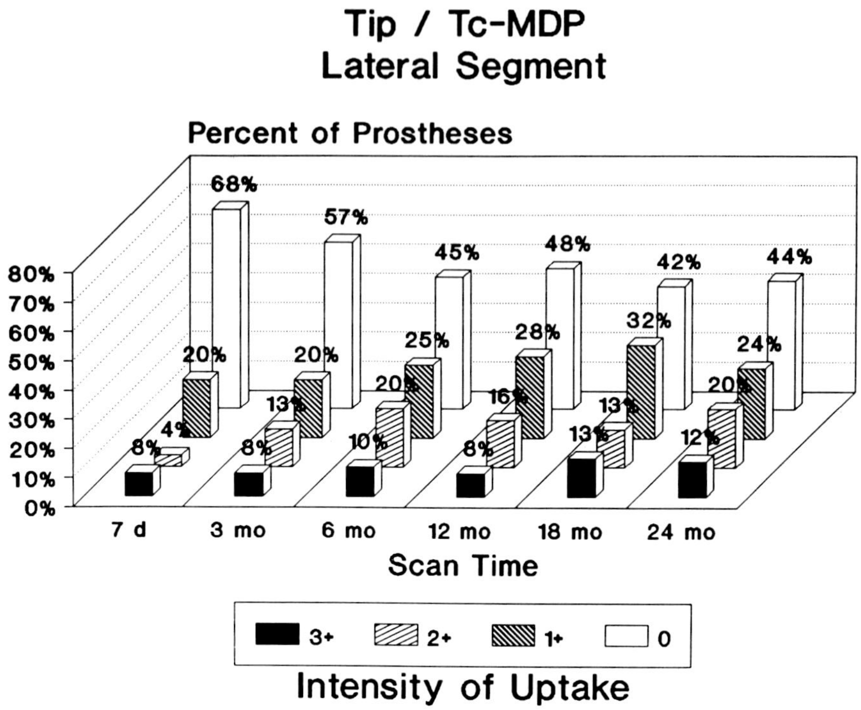

Figure 4.15. Trend in lateral segment activity.

The percentage of prostheses showing a trend in changing lateral segment Tc-MDP activity for a particular time interval. For example, during the interval encompassing 6 to 24 months postoperatively, 60% had stable or decreasing activity, 24% exhibited an increase in activity by one intensity grade, and increases by two and three intensity grades were each noted in 8%.
Comment: The overall trend with serial scanning is for activity to remain stable or decrease within the lateral segment. However, a closer look at Fig. 4.14 reveals that more hips demonstrated increased Tc-MDP activity in this region at 24 months than at 3 months. Increasing activity with time in the lateral or distal segment does not necessarily imply a complication.
(Reprinted with permission from the *Journal of Nuclear Medicine*; 1989;30:1321–1331; The Society of Nuclear Medicine.)

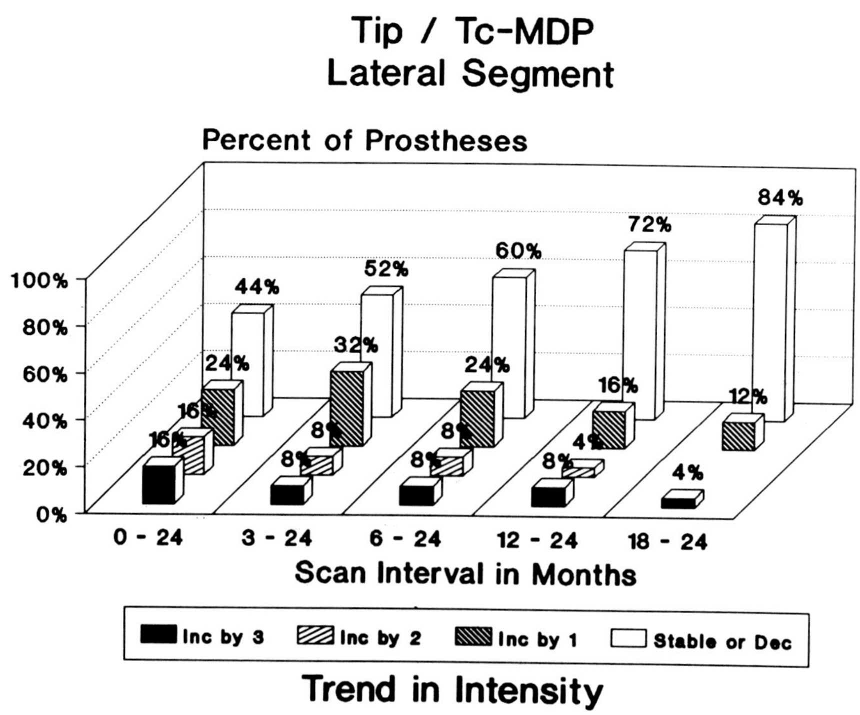

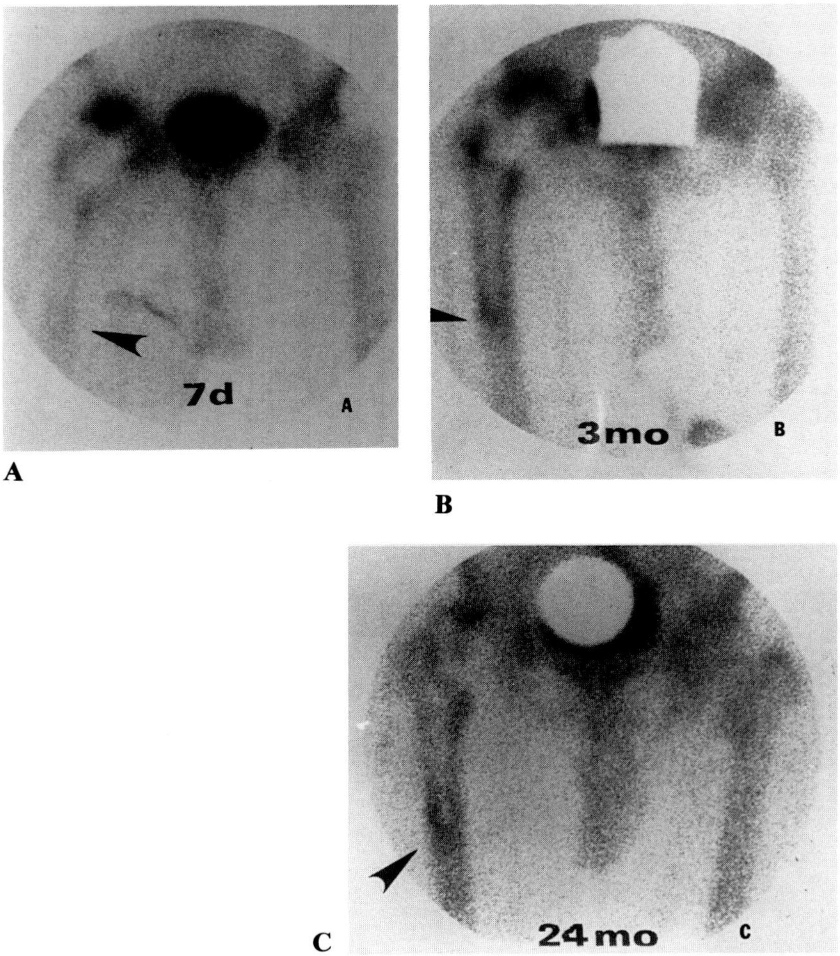

A

B

C

Figure 4.16. Example of changing tip activity with time.

Increasing tip activity (*arrowheads*) is noted from the 7-day scan (**A**) to the 3-month scan (**B**), then remained stable as demonstrated on the 24-month scan (**C**).

Figure 4.17. Example of changing tip activity with time.

Increasing tip activity (*arrowheads*) is noted from the 7-day scan (**A**) to the 12-month scan (**B**) to the 24-month scan (**C**). This activity also tends to become more lateral in location.

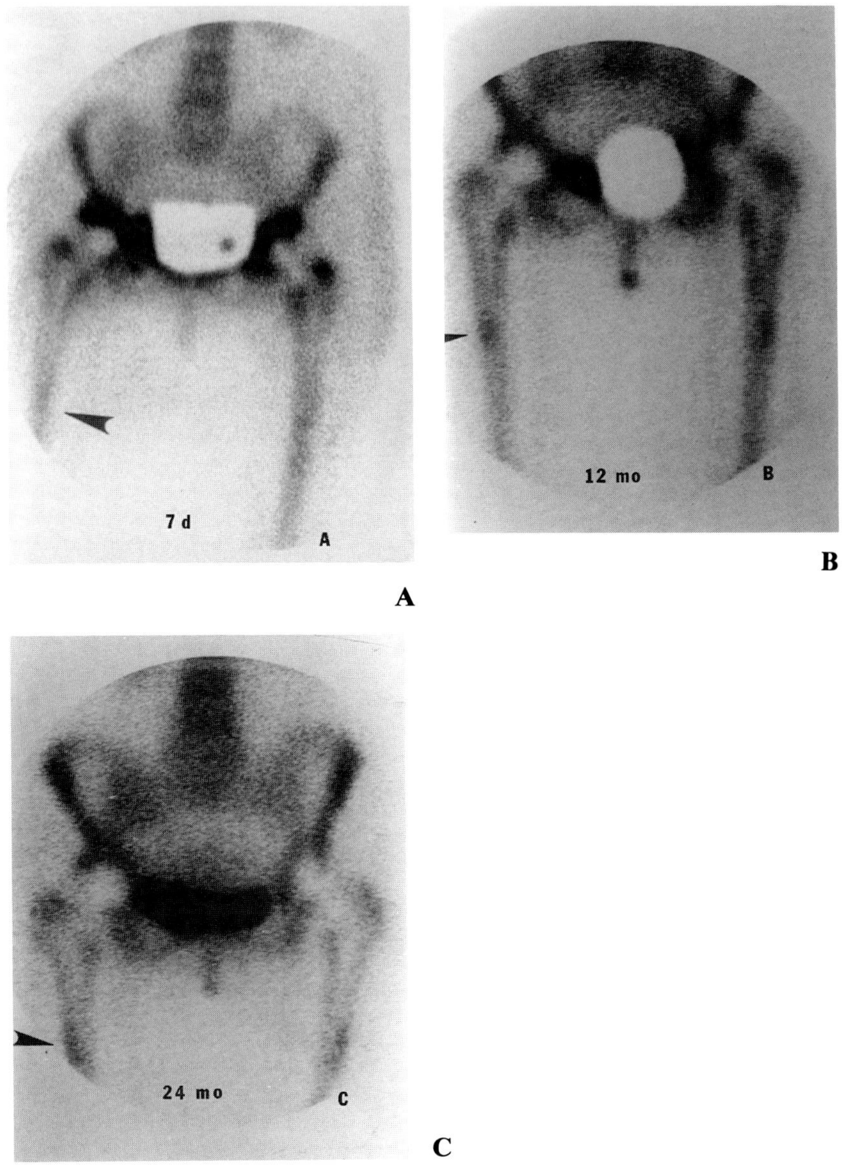

A B C

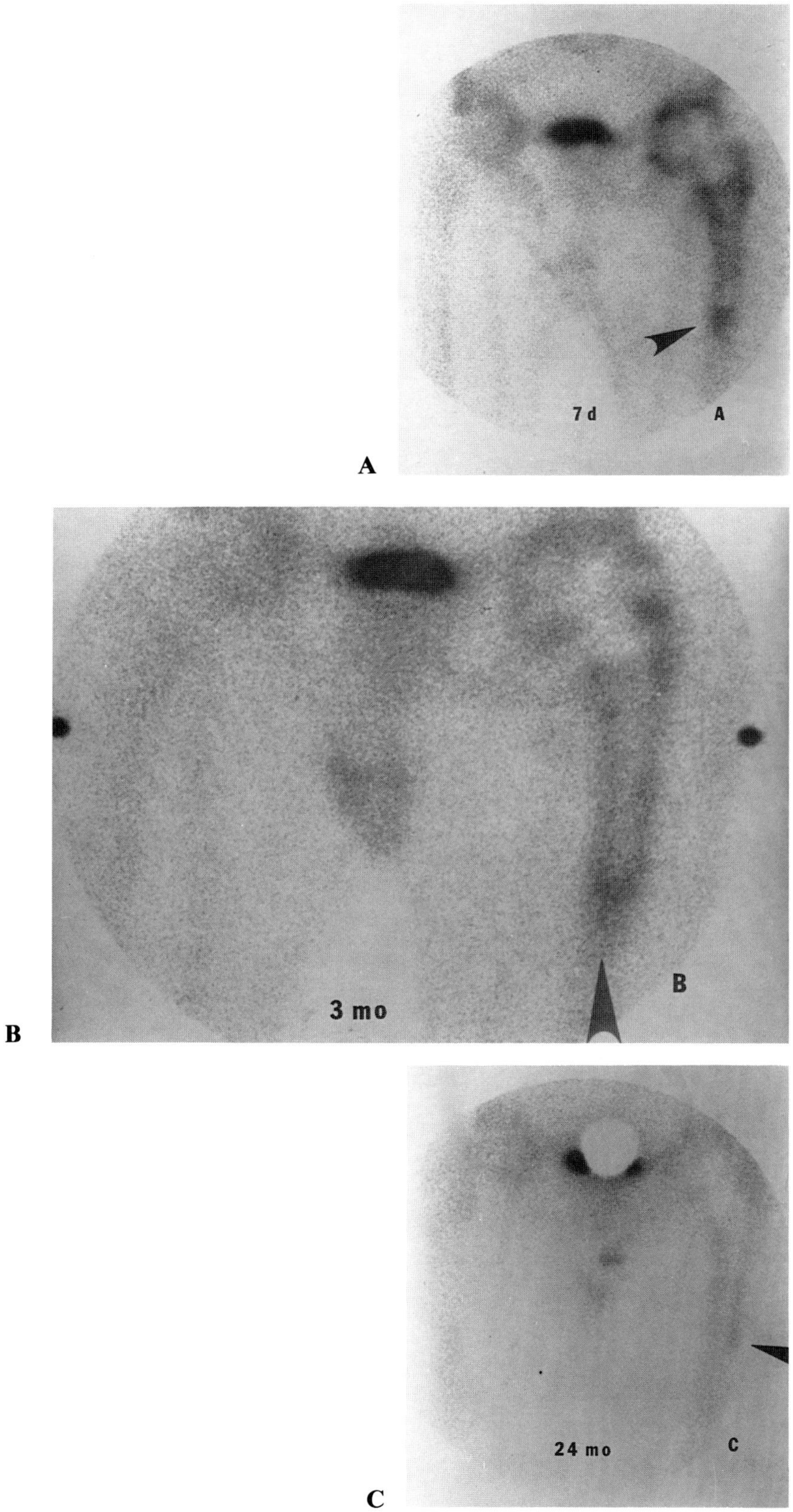

Figure 4.18. Example of changing location of tip activity.

This patient demonstrated "migrating" activity (*arrowheads*) from a more medial location on the 7-day scan (**A**) to a distal location on the 3-month scan (**B**), and finally to a lateral position on the 24-month scan (**C**).

Acetabulum

Flow and Blood Pool Study. Normal blood flow and blood pool in the acetabular region is noted. Refer to Figs. 4.3 and 4.5

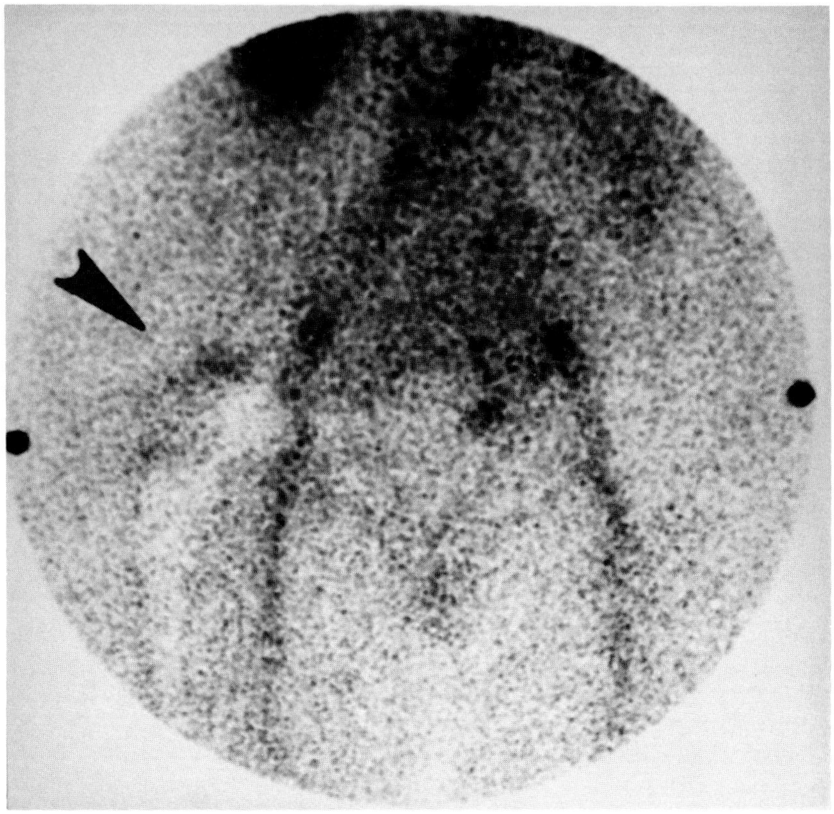

Figure 4.19. Increased acetabular blood pool.

Increased blood pool activity about the acetabulum is shown (*arrowhead*) on this 3-month postoperative scan in a patient with a right hip prosthesis.

Comment: Abnormal blood flow to the acetabular region was not seen in any of 134 flow studies. However, increased blood pool activity is not unusual, noted in 22% of 139 scans in our population. This was almost always confined to the first 3 postoperative months. Increased blood flow or abnormal blood pool activity beyond 3 months should be viewed with suspicion.

Bone Phase

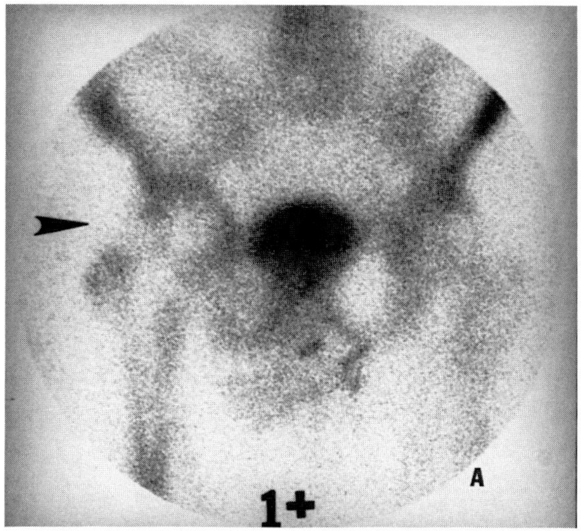

A

Figure 4.20. Examples of intensity grades of acetabular uptake.

The spectrum of Tc-MDP uptake in the acetabulum is shown. *Arrowheads* indicate the hip of interest. Grade 1+ (**A**) represented activity less than ipsilateral iliac crest, grade 2+ (**B**) equal to iliac crest, 3+ (**C**) greater than iliac crest, and 4+ (**D**) markedly greater than iliac crest. See Comment in Fig. 4.22.
(Reprinted with permission from the *Journal of Nuclear Medicine*; 1990;30:274–280; The Society of Nuclear Medicine.)

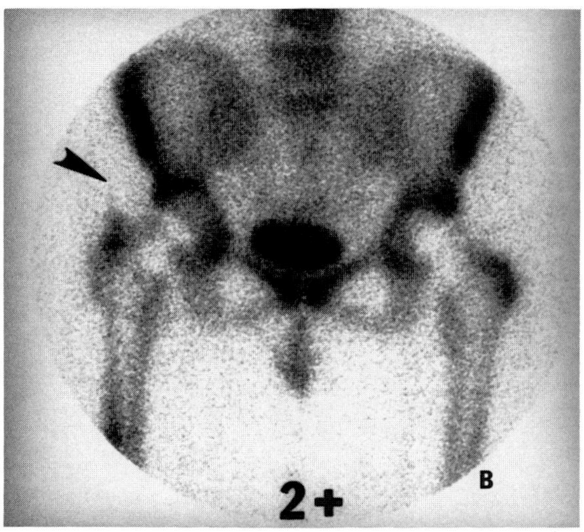

B

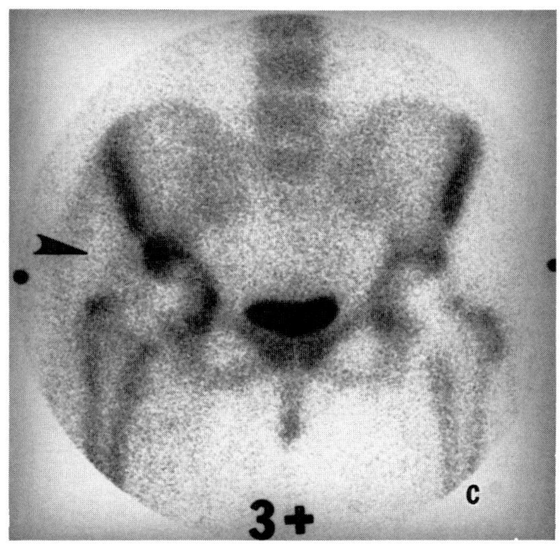

C

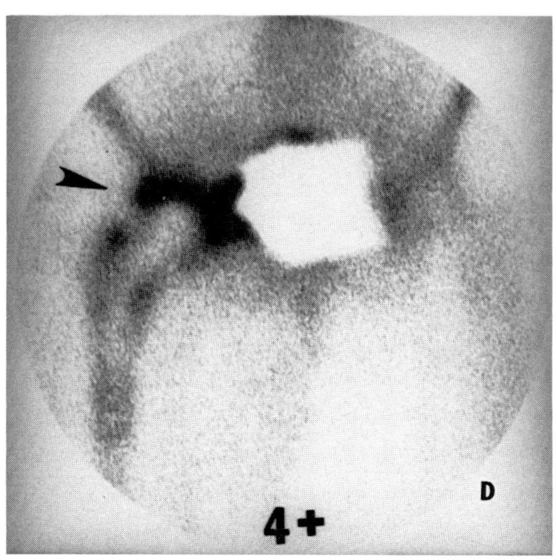

D

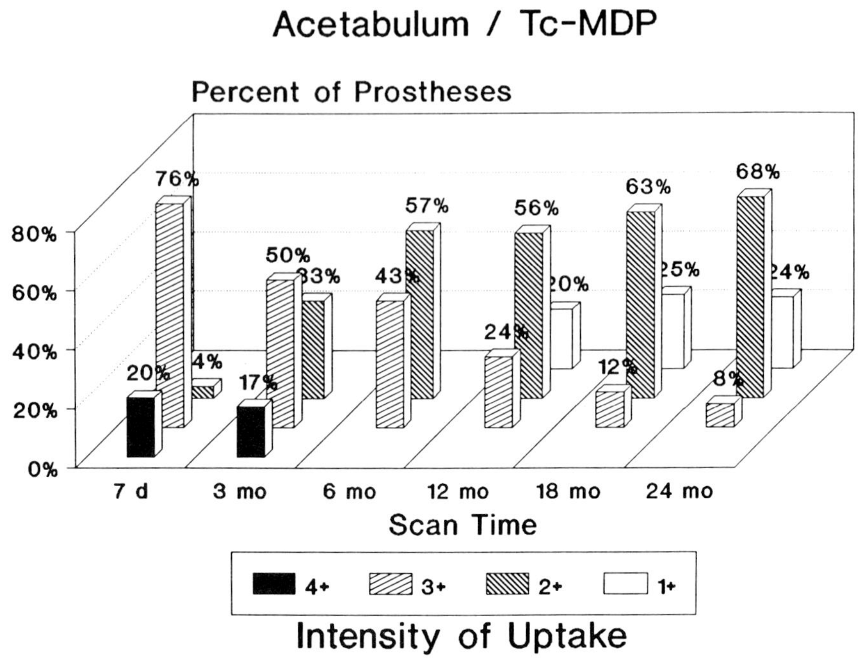

Figure 4.21. Acetabular activity.

The percentage of prostheses exhibiting a particular intensity of Tc-MDP uptake at a given scanning time. As time elapses from initial surgery, more prostheses demonstrate lower grades of uptake. See Comment in Fig. 4.22.
(Reprinted with permission from the *Journal of Nuclear Medicine*; 1990;31:274–280; The Society of Nuclear Medicine.)

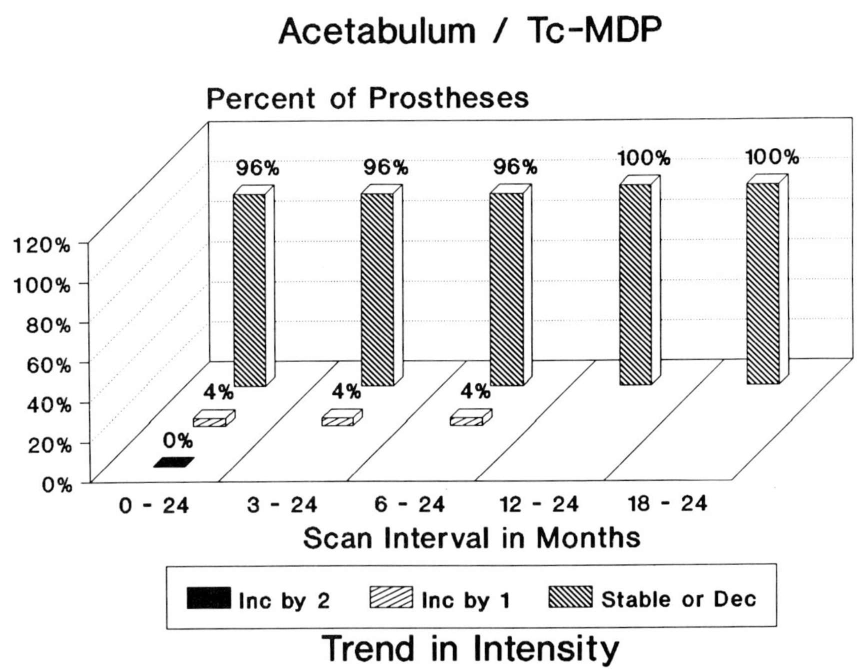

Figure 4.22. Trend in acetabular activity.

The percentage of prostheses manifesting a particular trend in changing Tc-MDP activity with serial scanning. For example, during the 6- to 24-month postoperative interval 96% of PCHA show stable or decreasing intensity of activity and only 4% had an increase by one intensity grade.
Comment: The presence of increased acetabular Tc-MDP uptake by itself is ubiquitous and has little significance. However, since activity almost invariably decreases or remains stable with time, any increase noted with serial scanning should raise suspicions of a complication. Again, having obtained a baseline scan may be extremely helpful in the interpretation of future scintigraphic studies. See Comment in Fig. 4.11. There would appear to be greater frequency of late uptake (1 or 2 years postoperatively) in porous coated arthroplasties than in cemented prostheses.
(Reprinted with permission from the *Journal of Nuclear Medicine*; 1990;31:274–280; The Society of Nuclear Medicine.)

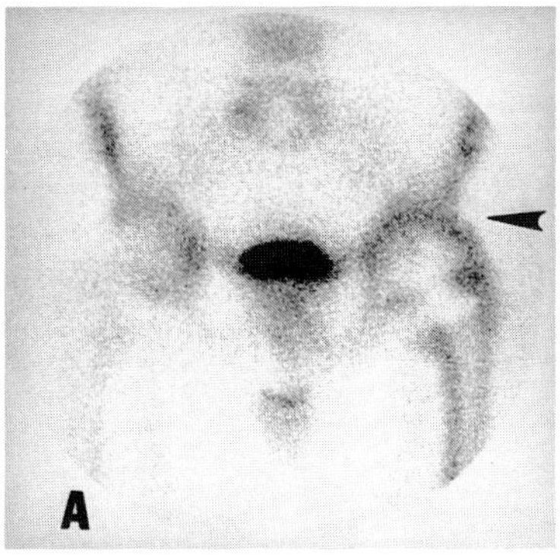

A

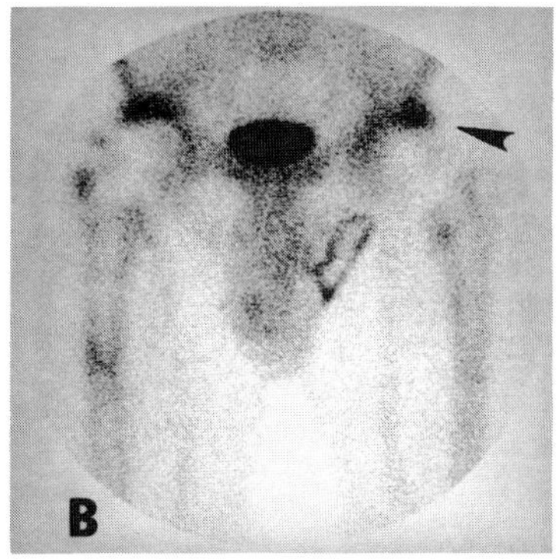

B

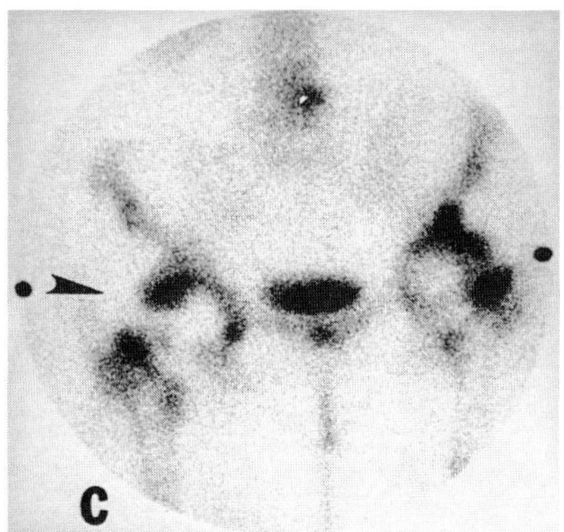

C

Figure 4.23. Patterns of acetabular activity.

Three patterns of Tc-MDP uptake commonly seen in our patient population are shown. *Arrowheads* indicate the hip of interest. Uniform uptake (**A**) was noted in 22% of our scans. In about half of the scans, greater intensity of uptake was noted in either the superior (**B**) or the inferior aspect of the acetabulum (*not shown*). In 25% of scans greater intensity of uptake was seen in both the superior and the inferior acetabulum (**C**).
(Reprinted with permission from the *Journal of Nuclear Medicine*; 1990;31:274–280; The Society of Nuclear Medicine.)

Figure 4.24. Examples of changing acetabular activity over time.

Decreasing activity in the left acetabulum (*arrows*) from the 7-day scan (**A**) to the 3-month scan (**B**) to the 24-month scan (**C**).

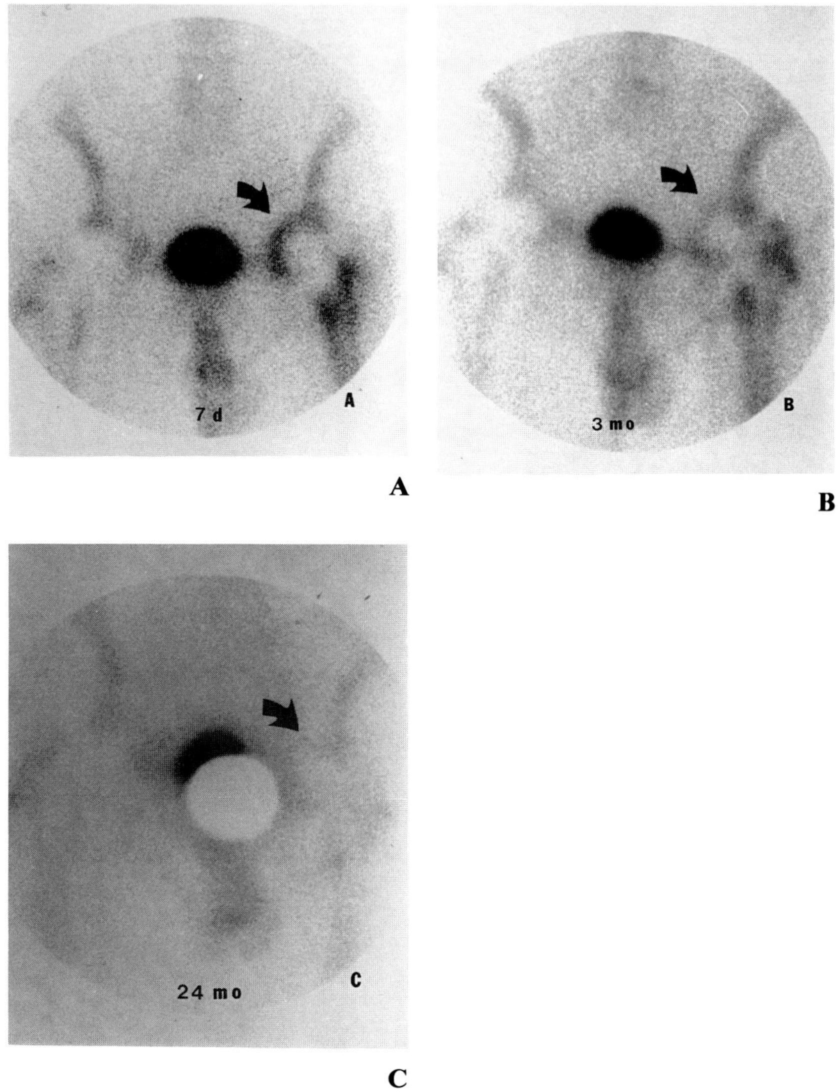

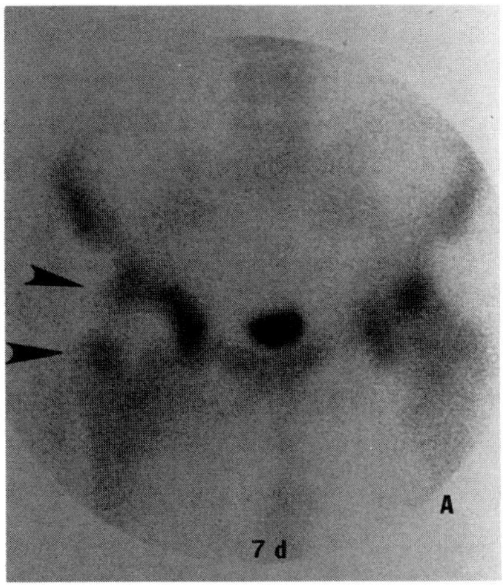

A

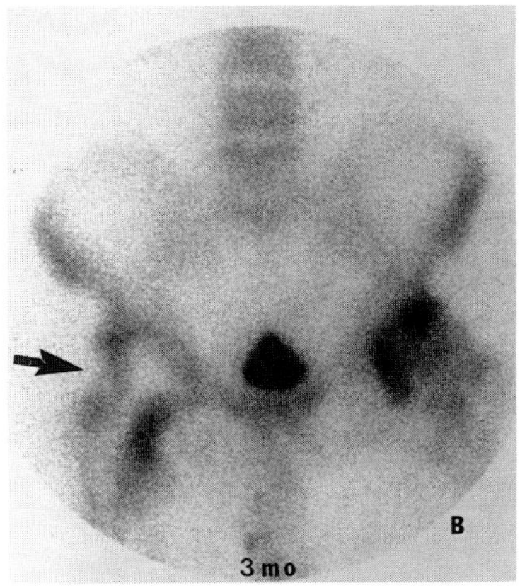

B

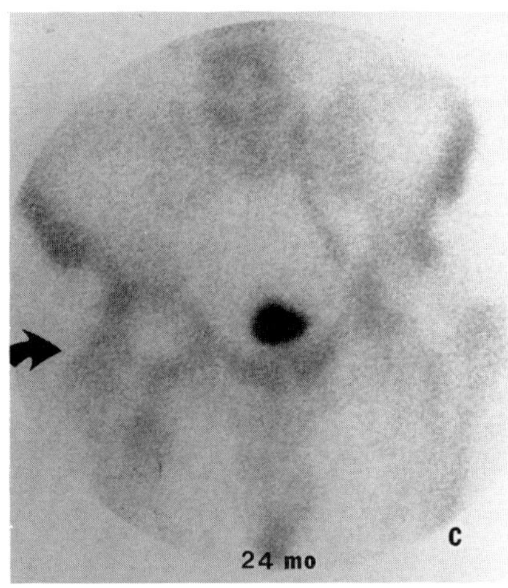

C

Figure 4.25. Uptake of Tc-MDP in heterotopic bone formation.

On the 7-day scan (**A**) increased activity is noted in the superior acetabulum and greater trochanter (*arrowheads*). Activity has extended into the soft tissues of the joint capsule (*straight arrow*) by 3 months (**B**) and completely "bridges" the joint (*curved arrow*) by 24 months (**C**). Heterotopic ossification was confirmed radiographically. Also note Fig. 4.23A. See Comment in Fig. 4.26.

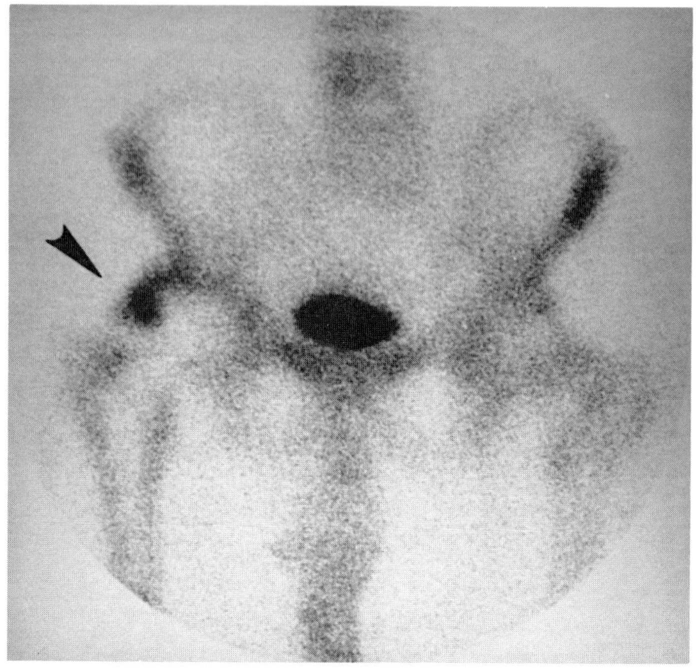

Figure 4.26. Uptake of Tc-MDP in heterotopic bone formation.

An intense focus of activity is noted on the lateral aspect of the right hip (*arrowhead*). Radiographic correlation indicated this was uptake in heterotopic ossification.
Comment: Increased uptake on bone scintigraphy should be correlated with radiographs to detect the possibility of Tc-MDP uptake in heterotopic ossification. Care should be taken to avoid interpreting this as indicative of prosthesis loosening or infection. We arbitrarily did not classify heterotopic bone formation as a complication for this study.

Trochanter

Flow and Blood Pool Study. Normal blood flow and blood pool in the trochanteric region are shown in Figs. 4.3 and 4.5.

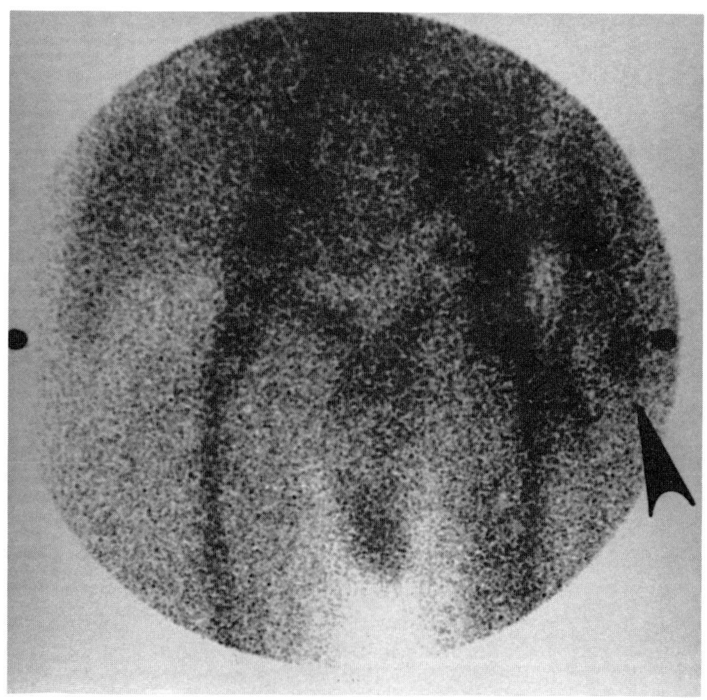

Figure 4.27. Increased blood pool activity in the trochanteric region is shown (*arrowhead*) in this scan performed 1 week after arthroplasty.

Comment: Abnormal blood flow to the trochanteric region was not seen in any of 135 flow studies. Increased blood pool activity was not infrequently noted (23% of scans in our series) but was generally confined to the first 3 postoperative months and never greater than 1+ in intensity. Increased blood flow at any time or increased blood pool activity beyond 3 months, especially if greater than 1+ in intensity, should be viewed with suspicion.

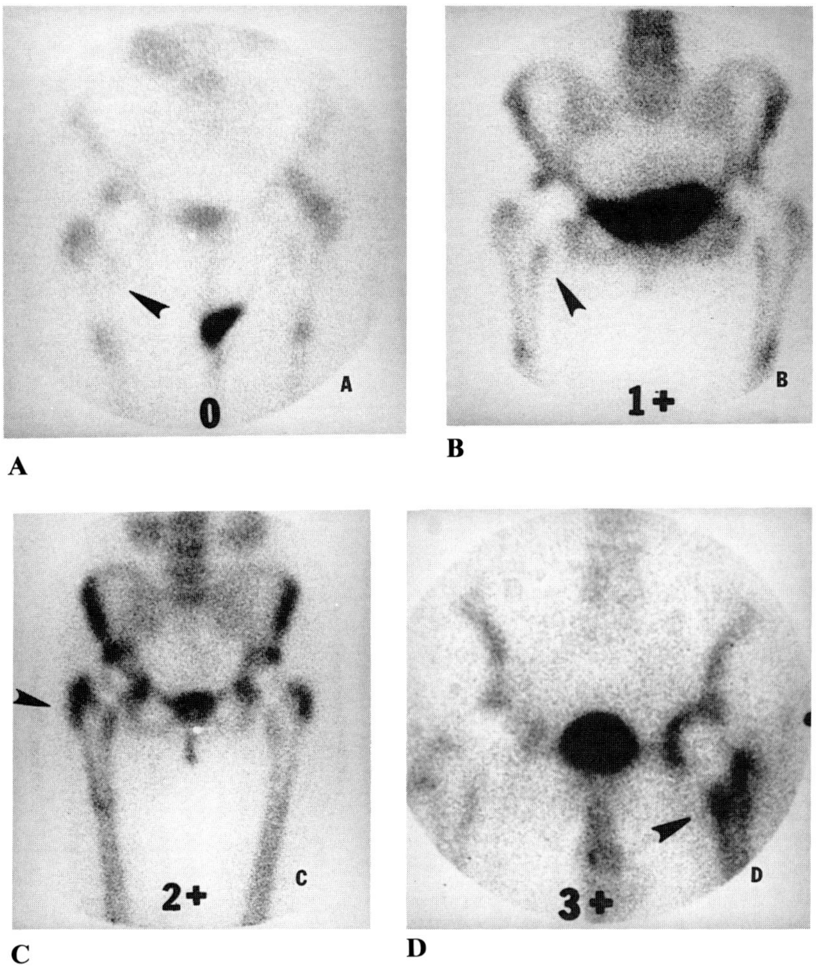

Bone Phase

Figure 4.28. Examples of intensity grades of trochanteric uptake.

The spectrum of Tc-MDP uptake in the trochanters is shown. *Arrowheads* indicate the region of interest. Grade 0 (**A**) represented activity equal to normal bone background (defined as uptake in normal femur), grade 1+ (**B**) was activity greater than background but less than iliac crest, grade 2+ (**C**) equal to iliac crest, and grade 3+ (**D**) greater than iliac crest.

Figure 4.29. Pattern of greater trochanter uptake.

Examples of Tc-MDP uptake in the greater trochanteric area are shown (*arrowheads*). **B** exhibits uptake that is more focal than **A**.

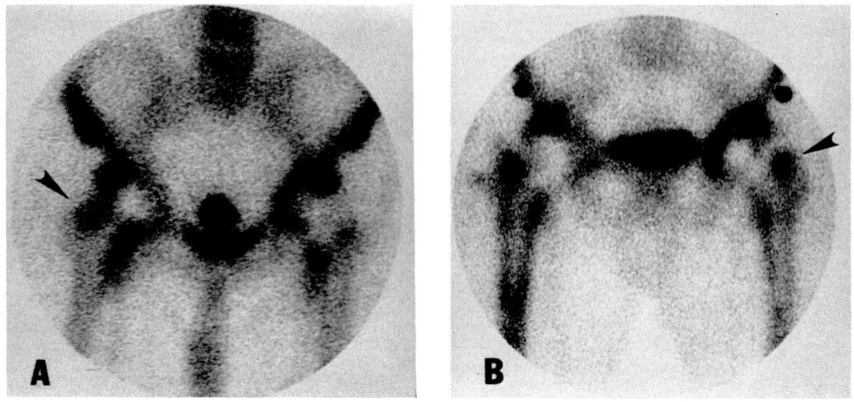

A B

Figure 4.30. Pattern of lesser trochanter uptake.

Linear Tc-MDP uptake in the lesser trochanteric (*arrowhead*) region is shown in this scan performed 1 year after arthroplasty.
Comment: Most prostheses in our study (94% of scans) demonstrated a linear pattern of Tc-MDP uptake at the lesser trochanter.

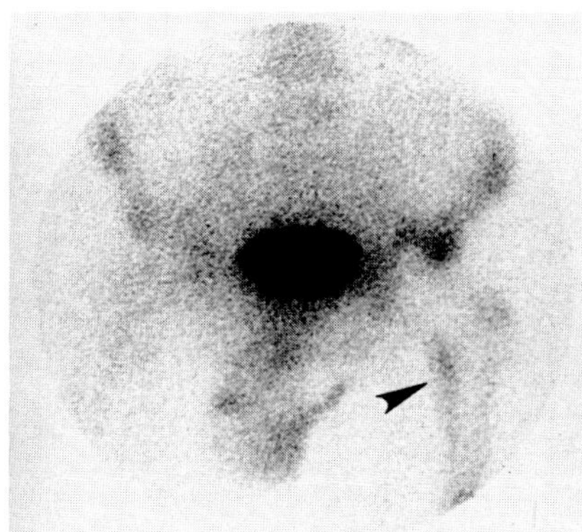

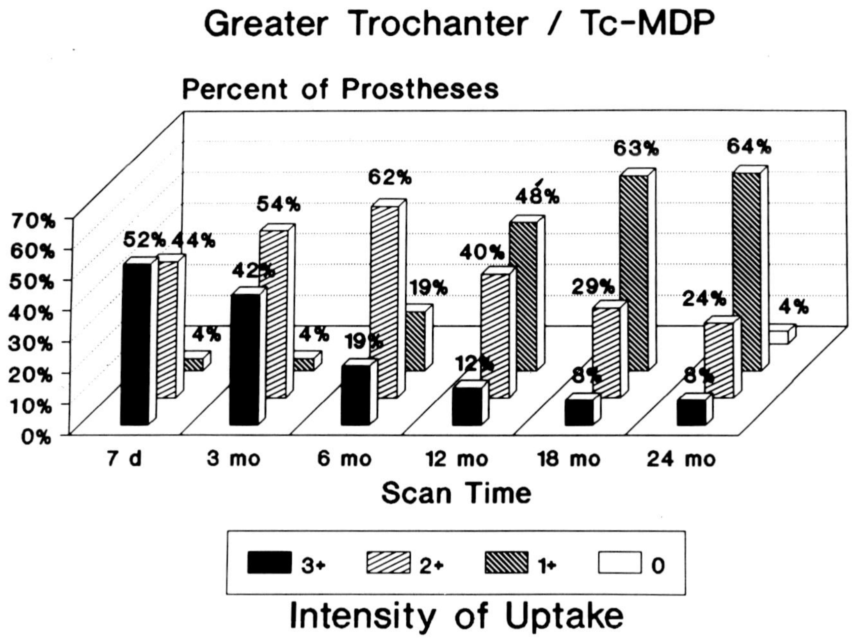

Figure 4.31. Greater trochanter activity.

The graph demonstrates the percentage of prostheses showing a given intensity of Tc-MDP uptake in the greater trochanter at the various scanning times. See Comment in Fig. 4.34.

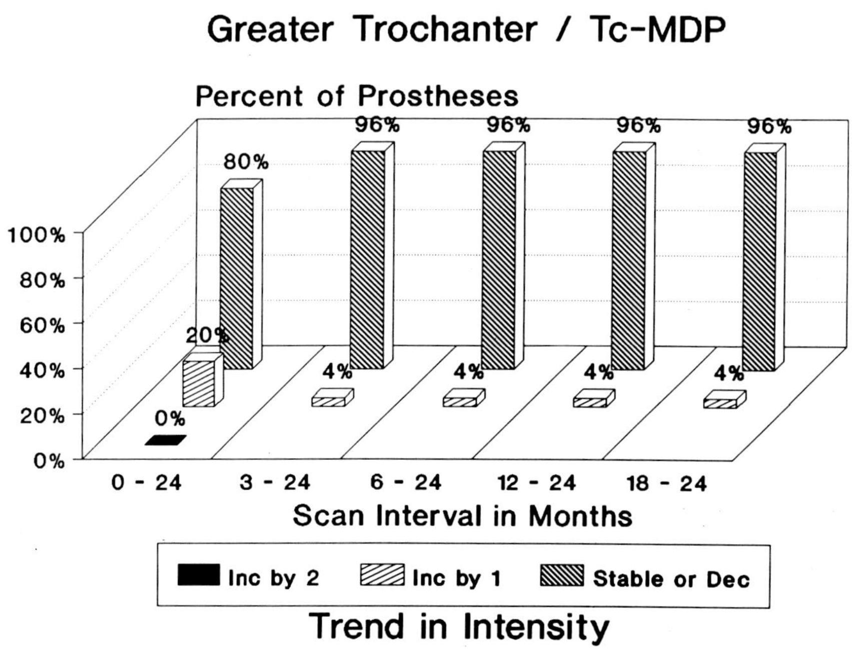

Figure 4.32. Trend in greater trochanter activity.

The percentage of prostheses demonstrating a trend in changing Tc-MDP intensity in the greater trochanter for a given time interval. For example, during the interval encompassing 3 to 24 months postoperatively, 96% of prostheses exhibited stable or decreasing activity and 4% showed an increase by one intensity grade. No prosthesis demonstrated an increase by two intensity grades during the study. See Comment in Fig. 4.34.

Figure 4.33. Lesser trochanter activity.

The percentage of prostheses demonstrating a given intensity of Tc-MDP uptake in the lesser trochanter at the various scanning times. See Comment in Fig. 4.34.

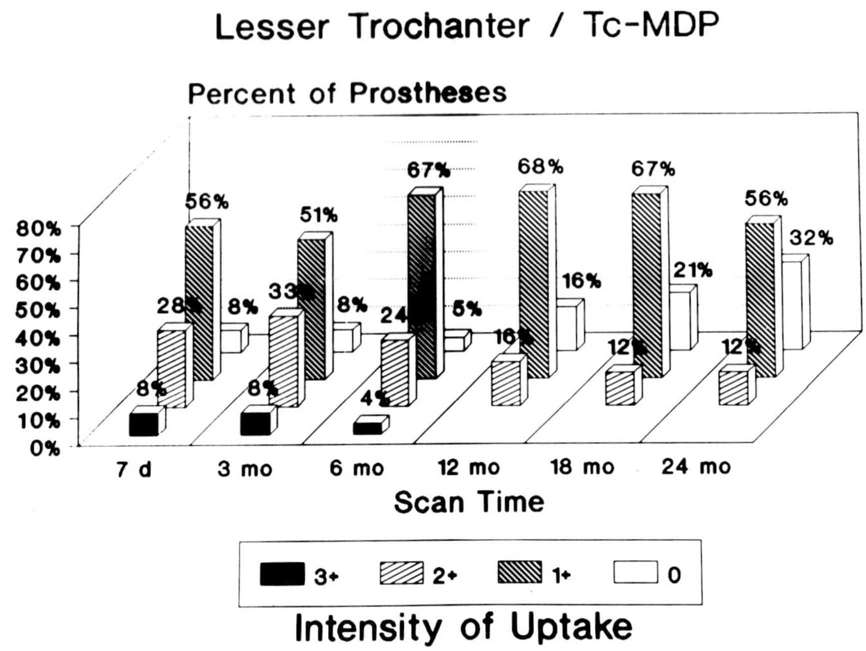

Figure 4.34. Trend in lesser trochanter activity.

The percentage of prostheses demonstrating a trend in changing Tc-MDP intensity in the lesser trochanter for a given time interval.

Comment: Increased Tc-MDP activity in the trochanters was common in our patient population, seen in 99% and 80% of scans in the greater and lesser trochanters, respectively. Persistence of significant activity at 24 months is more common in the greater trochanter and should not necessarily be interpreted as representing a complication. However, increasing uptake with time is unusual and should be viewed with concern.

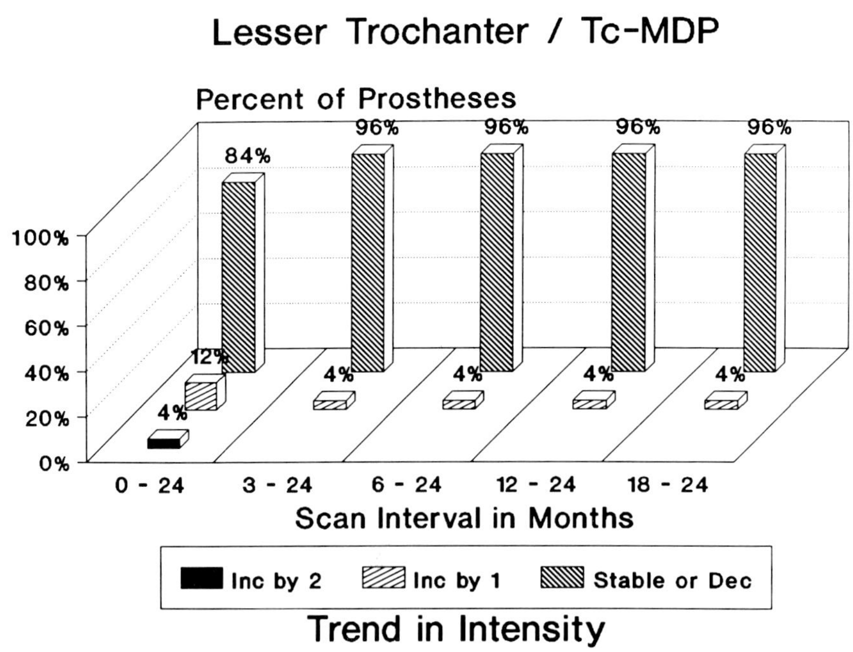

In-WBC Scintigraphy

Tip

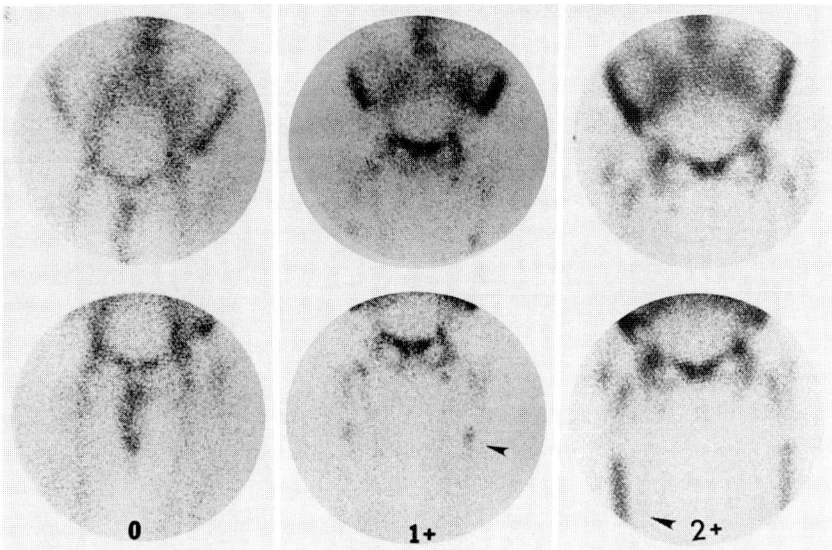

Figure 4.35. Examples of intensity grades of tip uptake.

Bottom row: The spectrum of increased tip uptake. Images over the pelvis for the same patient are shown immediately above so that comparison may be made with the iliac crest. The pelvic images were obtained on the same camera for the same length of time and at the same photographic intensity as the images of the prosthesis tip. Grade 0 represents activity less than or equal to background (defined as intensity of uptake in normal femur), grade 1+ is activity greater than background but less than iliac crest, and grade 2+ is defined as intensity approximately equal to the iliac crest. No prosthesis in our study exhibited tip uptake greater than iliac crest (grade 3+). *Arrowheads* indicate the side of interest.

Comment: In-WBC activity at the prosthesis tip was noted in 58% of scans and in 80% of all PCHA. The presence of In-WBC alone does not necessarily indicate the presence of infection.

(Reproduced with permission from the *Journal of Nuclear Medicine*; 1989;30:1321–1331; The Society of Nuclear Medicine.)

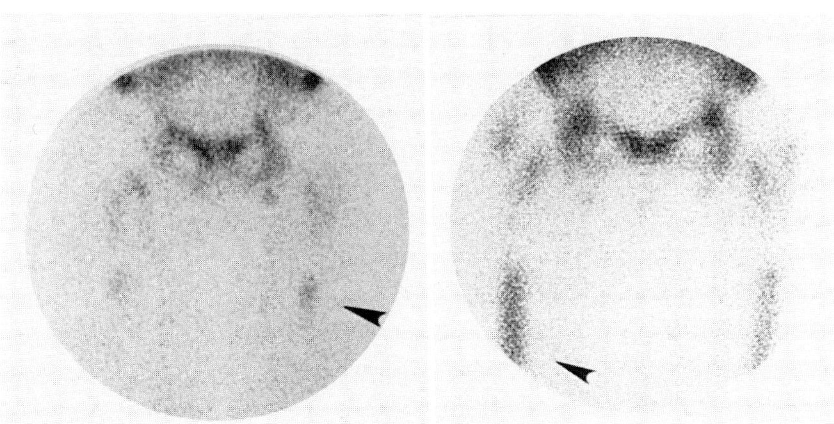

Figure 4.36. Patterns of In-WBC uptake.

The two patterns of In-WBC tip activity demonstrated in our patient population. *Left:* focal uptake is noted at the tip of a left PCHA (*arrowhead*). The other pattern (*right, arrowhead*) was of diffuse uptake extending from the tip into the distal femur in this patient with bilateral prostheses.

Comment: The focal and diffuse In-WBC uptake each occurred in approximately 50% of scans and PCHA. No change from one pattern to another was noted with serial scanning. In-WBC activity in a pattern other than these might suggest the presence of a complication.

(Reproduced with permission from the *Journal of Nuclear Medicine*; 1989;30:1321–3113; The Society of Nuclear Medicine.)

Figure 4.37. Example of changing In-WBC tip activity with time.

This patient demonstrates the diffuse pattern of In-WBC activity (*arrowheads*) decreasing over time. **A** was obtained 7 days, **B** at 12 months, and **C** at 24 months postoperatively.

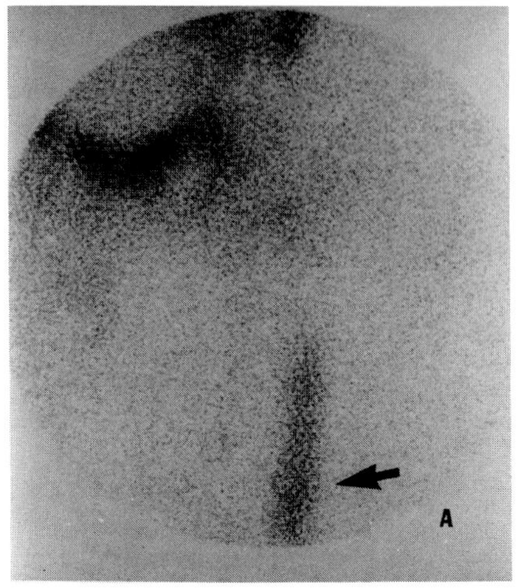

A

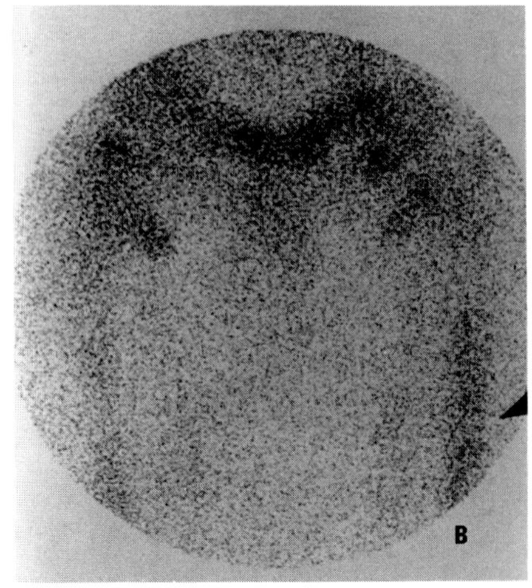

B

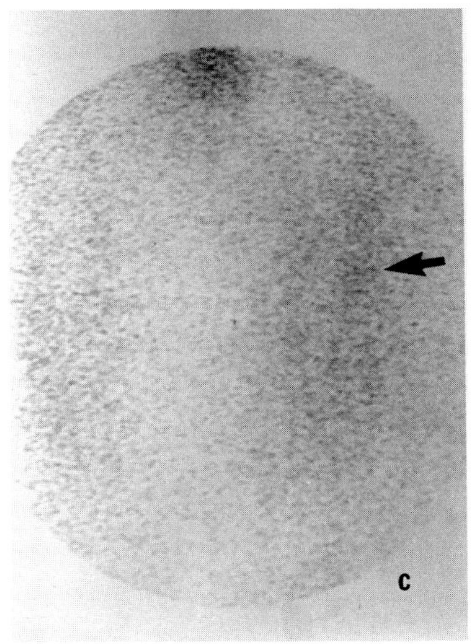

C

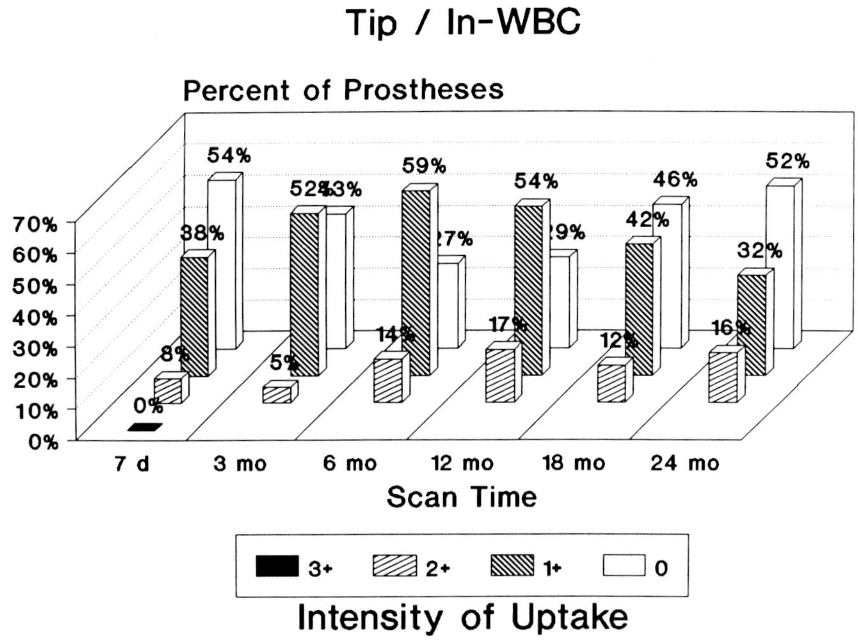

Figure 4.38. Tip activity.

The percentage of prostheses having a given intensity of In-WBC uptake at a particular scanning time. See Comment in Fig. 4.39. (Reprinted with permission from the *Journal of Nuclear Medicine*; 1989;30:1321–1331; The Society of Nuclear Medicine.)

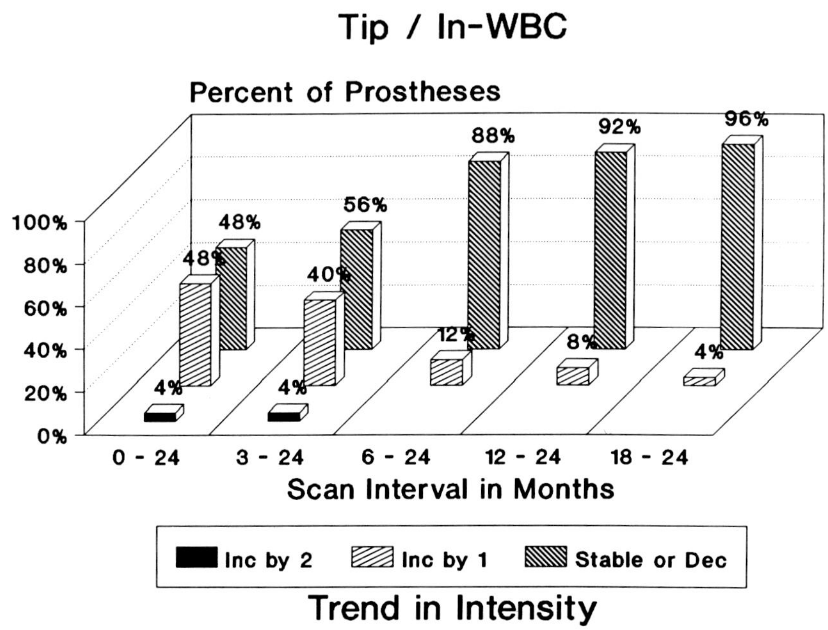

Figure 4.39. Trend in tip activity.

The percentage of prostheses exhibiting a trend in changing In-WBC activity with serial scanning. For example, during the time interval encompassing the 6th to the 24th month postoperatively, 88% of prostheses demonstrated stable or decreasing activity and 12% showed an increase in activity by one intensity grade.

Comment: Persistent In-WBC uptake at the prosthetic tip is not uncommon and its presence alone does not necessarily indicate an infection. However, with a few exceptions, those PCHA that did show In-WBC uptake typically demonstrated stable or decreasing activity with serial scanning. Intensity of In-WBC uptake greater than the iliac crest at any time or increasing uptake with time beyond the first 12 months postoperatively should raise the suspicion of a complication.

The relative intensity of uptake on the In-WBC scan was less than Tc-MDP uptake on the concurrent bone scan in 57% of scans, equal to Tc-MDP uptake in 28% of scans, and greater than Tc-MDP uptake in 15%.

(Reprinted with permission from the *Journal of Nuclear Medicine*; 1989;30:1321–1331; The Society of Nuclear Medicine.)

Acetabulum

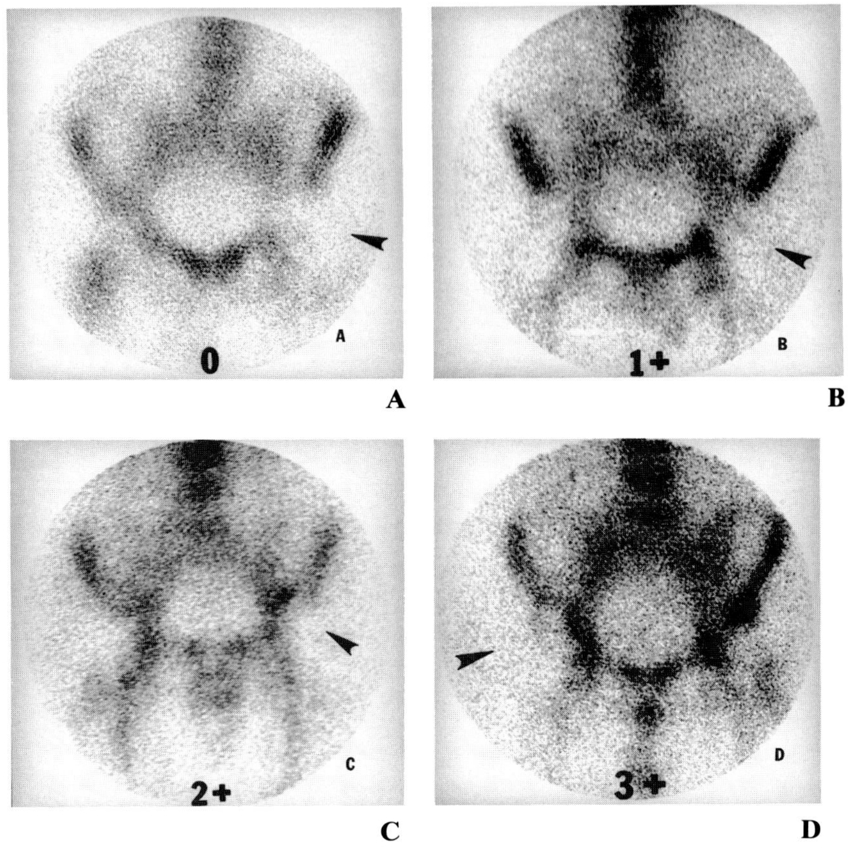

Figure 4.40. Examples of intensity grades of acetabular uptake.

The spectrum of In-WBC uptake in the acetabulum is shown. Grade 0 (**A**) represented activity less than or equal to background (defined as uptake in normal femur), grade 1+ (**B**) was greater than background but less than iliac crest, 2+ (**C**) equal to iliac crest, and 3+ (**D**) greater than iliac crest activity. *Arrowheads* indicate the hip of interest.
(Reprinted with permission from the *Journal of Nuclear Medicine*; 1990;31:274–280; The Society of Nuclear Medicine.)

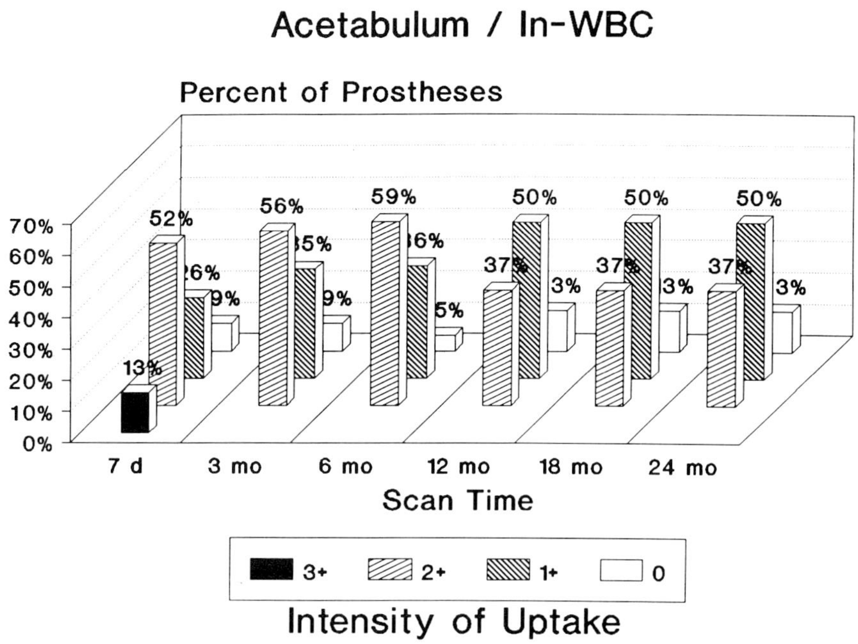

Figure 4.41. Acetabular uptake.

The percentage of prostheses having a particular intensity of In-WBC uptake at a given scanning time. See Comment in Fig. 4.42.

(Reprinted with permission from the *Journal of Nuclear Medicine*; 1990;31:274–280; The Society of Nuclear Medicine.)

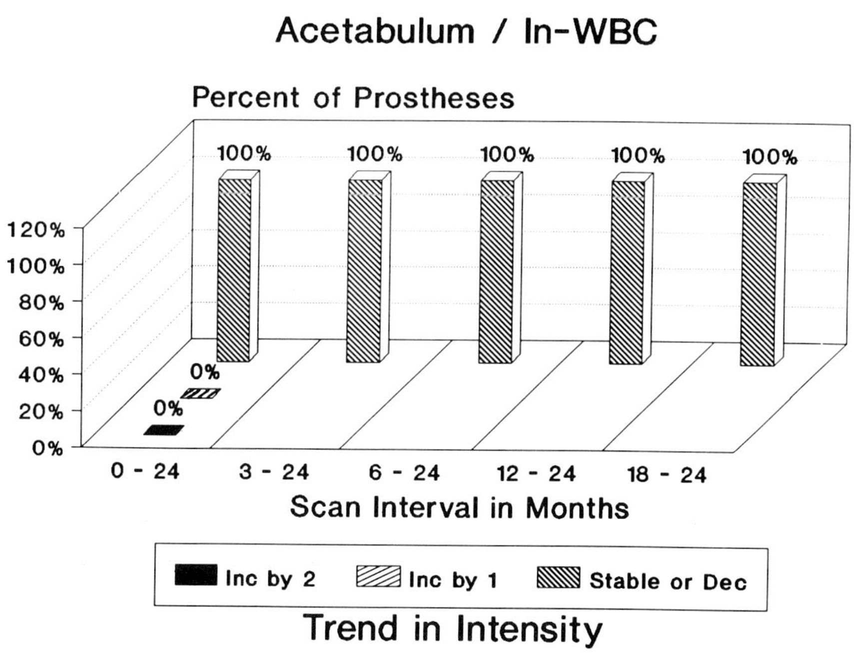

Figure 4.42. Trend in acetabular uptake.

The percentage of prostheses exhibiting a trend in changing intensity with serial scanning. All prostheses demonstrated stable or decreasing activity over time.

Comment: In-WBC uptake is extremely common with 90% of scans demonstrating uptake at some time postoperatively and with a considerable number still showing uptake equal to iliac crest (37%) at 24 months. Since stable or decreasing activity with time was the rule, however, any increase in uptake on a subsequent scan should be viewed with great suspicion.

Figure 4.43. Patterns of acetabular uptake.

Two distinct patterns of In-WBC activity are shown (*arrows*). Uniform acetabular activity was noted in 39% of scans and is demonstrated in **A**. Nonuniform uptake, typically characterized by decreased activity centrally and shown in **B**, occurred in 61% of scans.

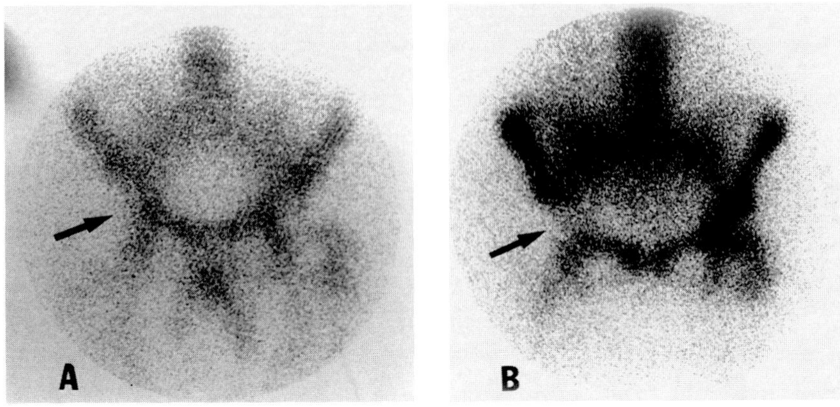

A B

Figure 4.44. In-WBC uptake in inguinal lymph nodes.

An example of multiple focal areas (*arrows*) of In-WBC uptake over the inguinal regions is shown in a patient with a right hip prosthesis.
Comment: This focal activity was noted in 37% of scans and in 60% of prostheses in the patients we studied. It did not correlate with the side of the prosthesis, the time since surgery, or with the presence of any symptoms. It is presumed to represent nonspecific uptake in lymph nodes and should not necessarily be interpreted as representing an abnormality.
(Reprinted with permission from the *Journal of Nuclear Medicine*; 1990;31:274–280; The Society of Nuclear Medicine.)

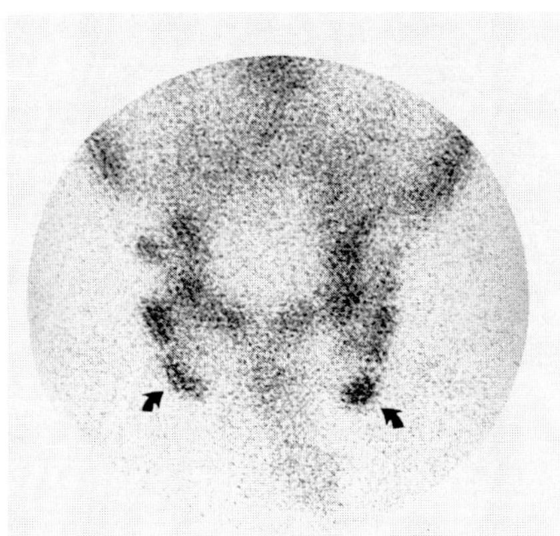

Trochanter

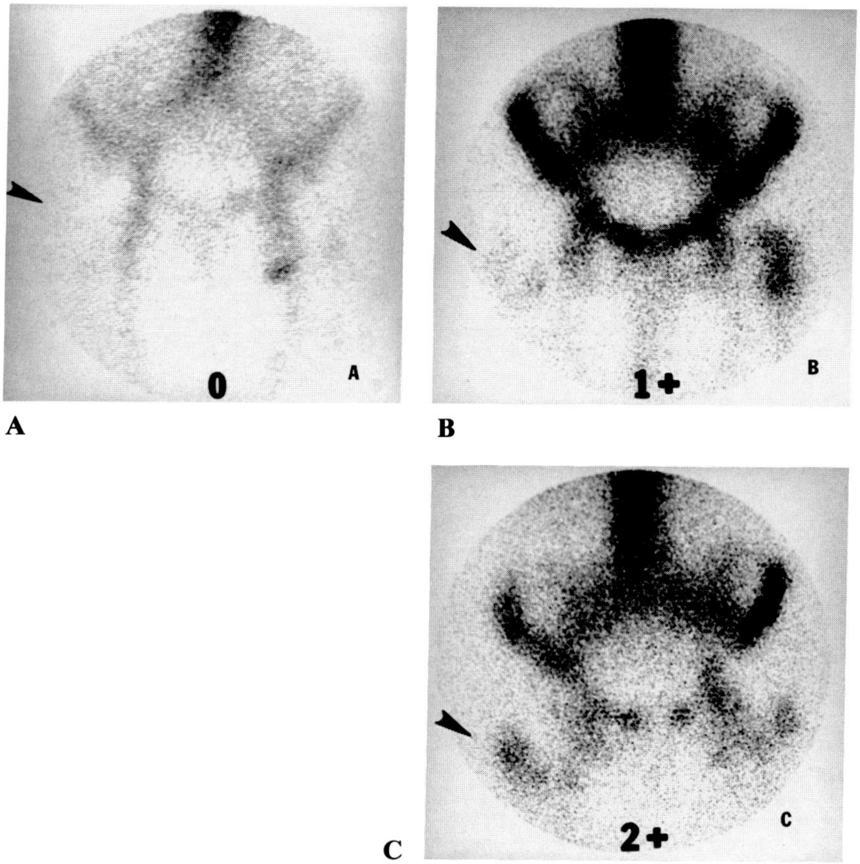

A B C

Figure 4.45. Example of intensity grades of trochanteric uptake.

The spectrum of In-WBC uptake in the region of the trochanters is shown. Grade 0 activity, represented by **A**, demonstrates activity equal to background (defined as uptake in normal femur). Grade 1+ is activity greater than background but less that iliac crest (**B**), and grade 2+ is equal to iliac crest (**C**). *Arrowheads* indicate the area of activity considered. No prosthesis demonstrated grade 3+ In-WBC uptake in the trochanteric area.

Figure 4.46. Intensity of uptake in greater trochanter.

The percentage of prostheses demonstrating a given intensity of In-WBC uptake in the greater trochanter at the various scanning times. See Comment in Fig. 4.49.

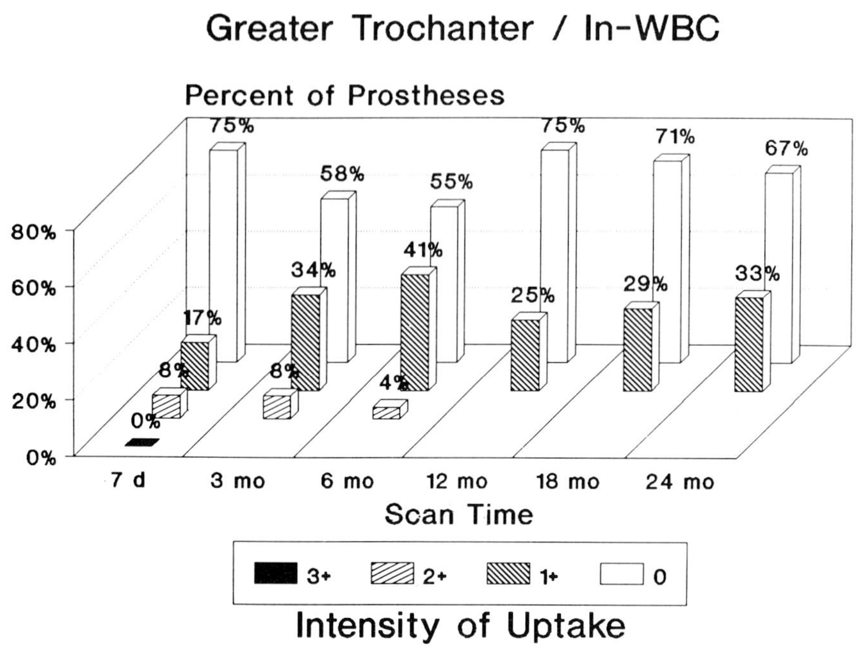

Figure 4.47. Trend in greater trochanter intensity.

The percentage of prostheses demonstrating a trend in changing In-WBC intensity in the greater trochanter for a given time interval. See Comment in Fig. 4.49.

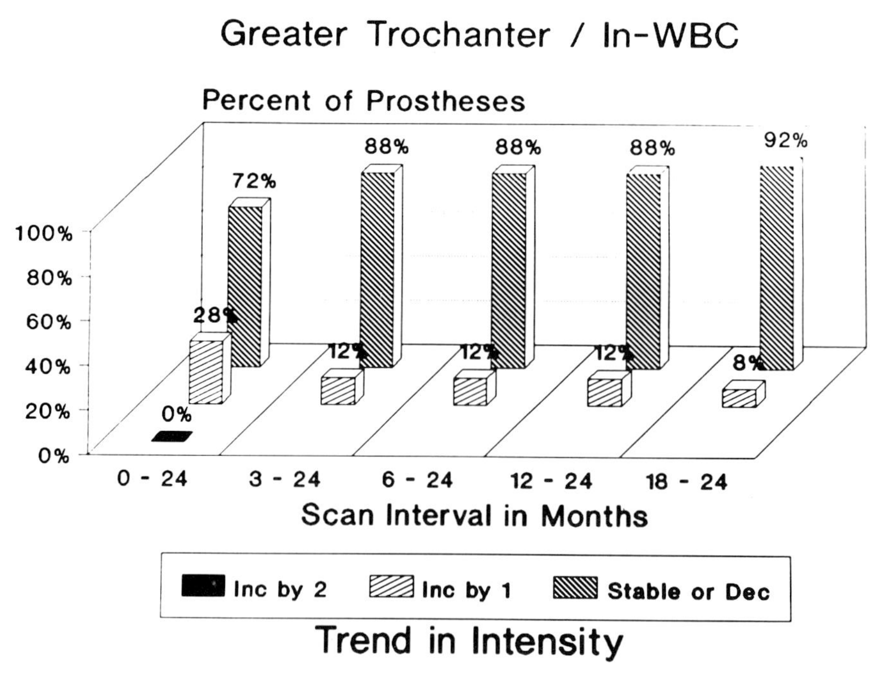

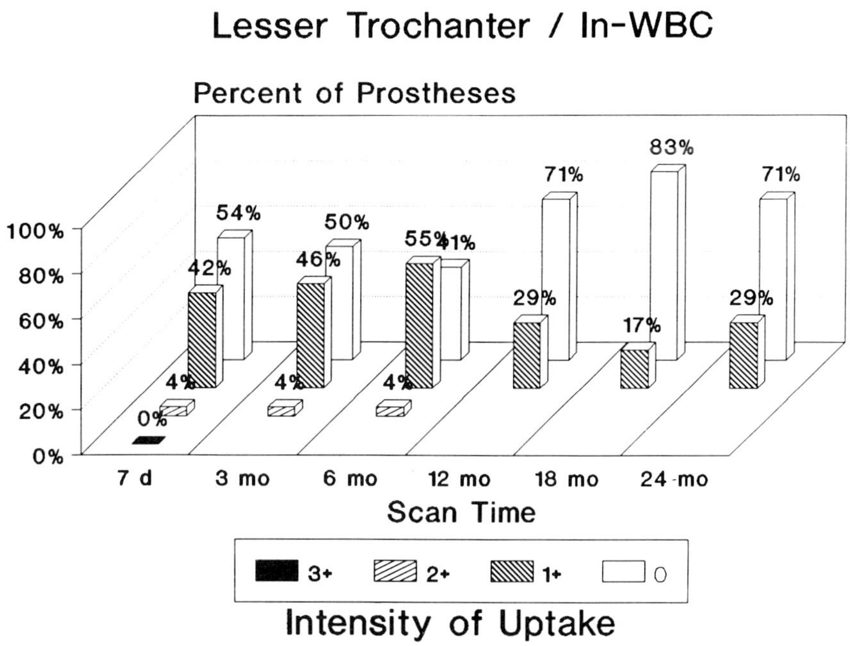

Figure 4.48. Intensity of uptake in lesser trochanter.

The percentage of prostheses demonstrating a given intensity of In-WBC uptake in the greater trochanter at the various scanning times. See Comment in Fig. 4.49.

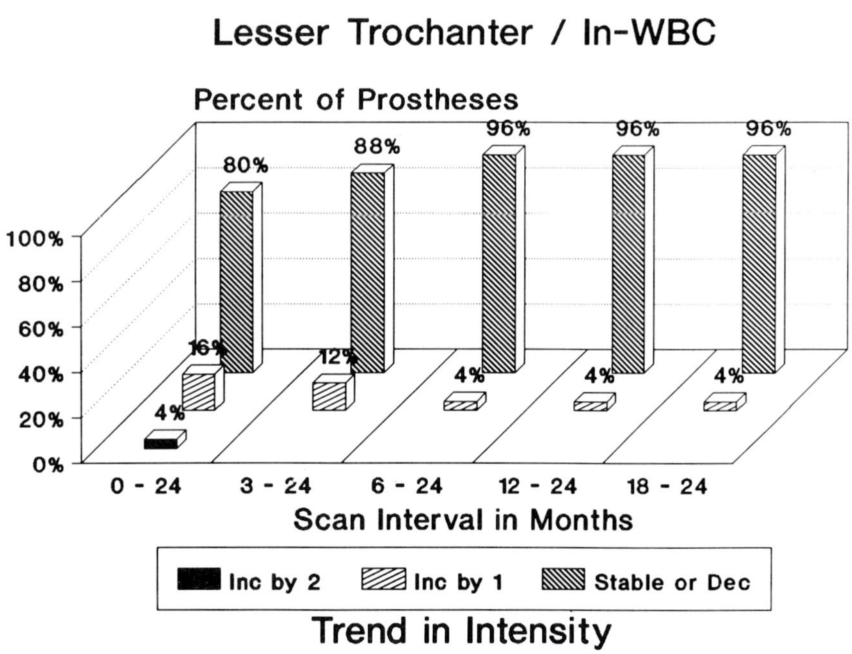

Figure 4.49. Trend in lesser trochanter intensity.

The percentage of prostheses demonstrating a trend in changing In-WBC intensity in the lesser trochanter for a given time interval.

Comment: Frequency of In-WBC uptake in the trochanteric region is common (34% and 42% of scans in the greater and lesser trochanters, respectively) and its presence alone does not necessarily represent infection. Any In-WBC intensity greater than iliac crest intensity should be viewed with caution. An increase in In-WBC intensity with serial scanning is not uncommon in the first 6 months postoperatively but beyond this time should be viewed with suspicion.

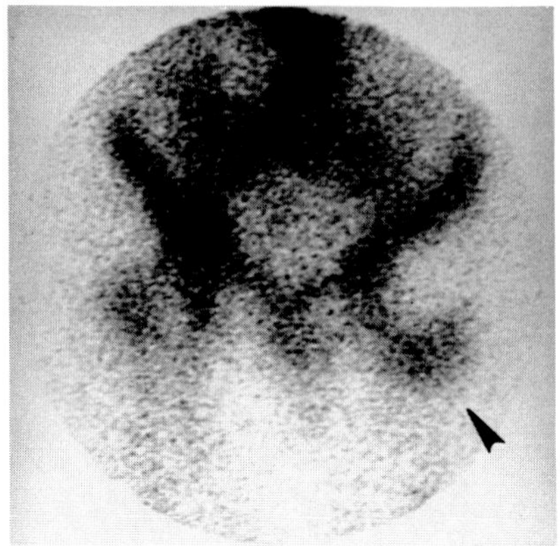

Figure 4.50. Intertrochanteric In-WBC uptake.

This prosthesis exhibited intertrochanteric In-WBC uptake (*arrowhead*) at 24 months postoperatively in the absence of any symptoms or signs of infection.

Comment: Even considerable In-WBC activity, without other corroborating evidence of infection, should be interpreted with caution. Correlation of uptake on In-WBC with marrow uptake on a technetium sulfur colloid bone marrow scan may be helpful in this regard.

References

1. Merkel KD, Brown ML, Fitzgerald RH. Sequential technetium-99m HMDP-gallium-67 citrate imaging for the evaluation of infection in the painful prosthesis. *J Nucl Med.* 1986;27:1413–1417.
2. Johnson JA, Christie MJ, Sandler MP, et al. Detection of occult infection following total joint arthroplasty using sequential technetium-99m HDP bone scintigraphy and indium-111 WBC imaging. *J Nucl Med.* 1988;29:1347–1353.
3. Magnuson JE, Brown ML, Hauser MF, et al. In-111-labeled leukocyte scintigraphy in suspected orthopedic prosthesis infection: Comparison with other imaging modalities. *Radiology.* 1988;168:235–239.
4. Utz JA, Lull RJ, Galvin EG. Asymptomatic total hip prosthesis: natural history determined using Tc-99m MDP bone scans. *Radiology.* 1986;161:509–512.
5. Haddad RJ, Cook SD, Thomas KA. Biological fixation of porous-coated implants. *J Bone Joint Surg.* 1987;69-A:1459–1466.
6. Oswald SG, Van Nostrand D, Savory CG, et al. Three phase bone scan and Indium white blood cell scintigraphy following porous coated hip arthroplasty: a prospective study of the prosthetic tip. *J Nucl Med.* 1989;30:1321–1331.
7. Oswald SG, Van Nostrand D, Savory CG, et al. The acetabulum: a prospective study of three phase bone and Indium white blood cell scintigraphy following porous coated hip arthroplasty. *J Nucl Med.* 1990;31:274–280.
8. Product literature insert. Amersham Corporation, 2636 South Clearbrook Dr., Arlington Heights, IL 60005.

Index